TO PROVIDE
SAFE PASSAGE:
THE HUMANISTIC
ASPECTS OF MEDICINE

TO PROVIDE SAFE PASSAGE: THE HUMANISTIC ASPECTS OF MEDICINE

edited by

Pauline L. Rabin, M.D.
*Associate Professor of Psychiatry,
Vanderbilt University*

and

David Rabin, M.D.
*Professor of Medicine and
Obstetrics and Gynecology,
Vanderbilt University*

Philosophical Library
New York

Library of Congress Cataloging in Publication Data

Main entry under title:

To provide safe passage.

1. Terminal care—Psychological aspects—Addresses, essays, lectures. 2. Long-term care of the sick—Psychological aspects—Addresses, essays lectures. 3. Death—Psychological aspects—Addresses, essays, lectures. 4. Physician and patient—Addresses, essays, lectures. I. Rabin, David. II. Rabin, Pauline L. [DNLM: 1. Physician-patient relations. 2. Attitude to Death. 3. Terminal care—Psychology. 4. Chronic disease—Psychology. 5. Death. W 62 T627]
R726.8.T6   1984   616'.029   84-4322
ISBN 0-8022-2462-8

For Grant W. Liddle
Physician, Scholar, Teacher, Humanist
and Cherished Friend

FOREWORD

John E. Chapman

Disease changes the human condition either abruptly or insidiously in ways over which the patient exercises little or no predictable control. As the changes emerge and are recognized, they are accompanied by profound emotional alterations which can influence the physical state. Physicians, in general, concentrate their efforts toward modifying favorably those processes of disease and injury which affect the human condition. Physicians are less comfortable when physical changes interlock with the emotional reactions they provoke and are uncertain how to facilitate accommodation. The hesitancy, sadness, and sense of defeat are all the more acute when therapy has failed or when the physician is faced with diseases which are usually called incurable. This volume comprises a collection of essays which discuss this most difficult segment of medical practice in a sensitive, authoritative manner. The contributors include a group of physicians with extensive experience with specific problems, as well as the perspective of the parents of a retarded child and the personal accounts of three patients. An important subtheme is the rather unique set of problems presented by the physician as patient. The interaction of physician, physician's illness, and physician colleagues represents a troika beset with mystique and opportunity as yet not addressed in a comprehensive manner. How can we formulate an understanding which provides opportunities and addresses the obstacles to successful interaction with ill colleagues? Five obstacles to change have been observed in the development of new nations and new organizations. These factors are not dissimilar to those faced by the physicians confronted by illness in a colleague.

(1) Excessive demands relative to time, energy, coping mechanisms, and circumstances.
(2) Inadequate resources for adapting to changing conditions, time, energy, and even attitude, but perhaps most important under stressful circumstances is inflexibility in reordering priorities.
(3) Isolation and division—the old relationship is lost and a new base of mutual support is not formed. All parties face a new isolation from a routine that formerly was comfortable and successful.
(4) Poor management—time, effort, and priority are all focused on short-term goals. A type of trivialization occurs such that the whole becomes the

simple sum of the parts, and the parts become smaller and smaller. The manager becomes the managed.

(5) Excessive traditionalism—we rely on the past as a guide to the future. When illness strikes, the past is, of course, not a reliable guide. A change in the health of a colleague who continues to function as a physician provokes anxiety, and one cannot fall back on tradition. The future becomes the traditional.

It is through understanding that we can convert obstacles into opportunity. The accounts represented by physicians of their own illness and its impact on every phase of life complements our understanding. Physicians have the understanding of the changes in the physiology, anatomy, and mechanism of injury and illness, but what of the changes in the patient as person? That is what the thoughts which follow are all about.

TABLE OF CONTENTS

Foreword
JOHN E. CHAPMAN   vii

Contributing Authors   xv

Acknowledgments   xix

Preface
DAVID RABIN AND PAULINE L. RABIN   xxi

The Care of the Patient
FRANCIS W. PEABODY   1

The Care of the Patient:
Francis Peabody Revisited
PAULINE L. RABIN AND DAVID RABIN   22

Compounding the Ordeal of ALS:
Isolation from My Fellow Physicians
DAVID RABIN, PAULINE L. RABIN, AND
RONI C. RABIN   29

The Pariah Syndrome:
The Social Disease of Chronic Illness
  DAVID RABIN AND PAULINE L. RABIN   38

Credo for Creeping Paralysis:
Cogito Ergo Sum
  PAULINE L. RABIN AND RONI C. RABIN   48

Chemotherapy from an Insider's Perspective
  KENNETH H. COHN   54

Anger as Freedom
  JORY GRAHAM   65

Doctors and Cancer Patients
  NATHAN SCHNAPER, TAMAR K. KELLNER, AND
  BARBARA KOEPPEL   80

The Hospice Concept
  IRIS KOZIL   97

The Management of Intractable Pain
  JOHN M. MERRILL   109

The Physician's Attitude toward Mental Illness
  MARC H. HOLLENDER   117

The Care of the Demented Patient
  CHARLES E. WELLS   133

The Mentally Retarded:
A Need for Understanding
  HOWARD COHEN AND JANE COHEN   143

Counseling and Support for Families with
Genetic Diseases
ANN P. GARBER AND DAVID L. RIMOIN   150

What Can I Do for a Dying Friend?
DAVID RABIN AND PAULINE L. RABIN   164

Death and Dying
PATRICK B. FRIEL   167

Acute Grief
PAULINE L. RABIN AND J. KIRBY PATE   185

Reflections on Medical Education
GODFREY S. GETZ   194

Some Reflections on Humanism in Medicine
ROSCOE R. ROBINSON AND F. TREMAINE BILLINGS   209

A Philosopher Reflects:
A Play against Night's Advance
RICHARD M. ZANER   222

Index   247

CONTRIBUTING AUTHORS

F. Tremaine Billings, M.D.
  Clinical Professor of Medicine Emeritus
  Vanderbilt University
  Nashville, Tennessee

John E. Chapman, M.D.
  Dean of Medicine, Vanderbilt University
  Nashville, Tennessee

Howard Cohen
  Baltimore, Maryland

Jane Cohen
  Baltimore, Maryland

Kenneth H. Cohn, M.D.
  Harvard Surgical Service
  New England Deaconess Hospital
  Boston, Massachusetts

Patrick B. Friel, M.D.
  Director of Consultation Liaison Psychiatry
  St. Francis Hospital
  Assistant Professor of Psychiatry
  University of Connecticut School of Medicine
  Hartford, Connecticut

Ann P. Garber, dr P.H.
  Director of Genetic Counselling
  Cedars-Sinai Medical Center
  Los Angeles, California

Godfrey S. Getz, M.D., Ph.D.
  Professor of Pathology and Biochemistry
  University of Chicago
  Chicago, Illinois

*Jory Graham
  Newspaper Columnist and Author

Marc H. Hollender, M.D.
  Professor of Psychiatry Emeritus, Vanderbilt University
  Nashville, Tennessee

Tamar K. Kellner
  Research Assistant
  Private Practice in Group Therapy
    for Cancer Patients and Family
  Baltimore, Maryland

Barbara Koeppel
  Freelance writer
  New York, New York

Iris A. Kozil
  Executive Director, Alive-Hospice of Nashville, Inc.
  Nashville, Tennessee

John M. Merrill, M.D.
Associate Professor of Medicine
Northwestern University Medical School
Chicago, Illinois

J. Kirby Pate, M.D.
Assistant Clinical Professor of Psychiatry
Vanderbilt University
Nashville, Tennessee

*Francis W. Peabody, M.D.
Professor of Medicine, Harvard Medical School
Boston, Massachusetts

David Rabin, M.D.
Professor of Medicine and Obstetrics-Gynecology
Vanderbilt University
Nashville, Tennessee

Pauline L. Rabin, M.D.
Associate Professor of Psychiatry, Vanderbilt University
Nashville, Tennessee

Roni Rabin
Education Reporter, The Nashville Banner
Nashville, Tennessee

David L. Rimoin, M.D., Ph.D.
Professor of Medicine and Pediatrics
Chief, Division of Medical Genetics
Harbor-UCLA Medical Center
Torrance, California

Roscoe R. Robinson, M.D.
Vice-Chancellor for Medical Affairs
Professor of Medicine, Vanderbilt University
Nashville, Tennessee

Nathan Schnaper, M.D.
  Professor of Psychiatry and Oncology
  University of Maryland School of Medicine
  Head, Psychiatry Section
  University of Maryland Cancer Center
  Baltimore, Maryland

Charles E. Wells, M.D.
  Professor of Psychiatry and Neurology
  Vanderbilt University
  Nashville, Tennessee

Richard M. Zaner, Ph.D.
  Ann Geddes Stahlman Professor of Medical Ethics
  Department of Medicine, Vanderbilt University
  Nashville, Tennessee

*deceased

ACKNOWLEDGMENTS

The editors wish to acknowledge kind permission to reprint the following articles appearing in this volume:

"The Care of the Patient" by Francis W. Peabody. The Journal of the American Medical Association, March 19, 1927, volume 88, pages 877-882. Copyright 1927, American Medical Association.

"Francis Peabody Revisited" by Pauline L. Rabin and David Rabin. The Journal of the American Medical Association, August 10, 1984, volume 252, pages 819-820. Copyright 1984, American Medical Association.

"Compounding the Ordeal of ALS: Isolation from My Fellow Physicians" by David Rabin, Pauline L. Rabin, and Roni C. Rabin. The New England Journal of Medicine, volume 307, pages 506-509, 1982.

The editors wish to thank Ms. Patty Adams and Ms. Bettye Ridley for their unstinting help in the preparation of this volume.

PREFACE

David Rabin and Pauline L. Rabin

Much is expected of the physician. He should be knowledgeable, he should be skillful, he should be articulate, and he should have a good bedside manner. The body of knowledge which he is required to master is fomidable. The technical procedures with which he must be familiar grow at an increasing pace. The therapeutic drugs which he may be required to use but must never abuse seem to be infinitely complex. The medical literature, research and clinical, with which he must keep abreast is voluminous. The student embarking upon a medical education in this era of high technology is intimidated by the enormity of the factual information and skills subtended by the physician's domain. It is hardly surprising that those lectures devoted to humanity and compassion are often undervalued or considered redundant and unnecessary. These qualities are considered indivisible from the choice of medi-

cine as a career. Perhaps they are. However, the burden
of acquiring sufficient knowledge in the basic sciences
programs the physician to respect factual knowledge
and crowds out the broader horizons of the medical
profession. The physician engaged in a rigorous and
exhaustive clinical practice is required to take a history, complete a physical examination, send off the
blood samples, and check on the laboratory results. In
all this frenetic activity, the patient's pain, suffering,
fear, and isolation may be overlooked. The result is
often an emphasis on *the disease process*.

Without in any sense decrying technological accomplishments in the treatment of the acutely ill and in
improving the adaptation of the chronically ill, here it
is our purpose to focus and emphasize the human
aspects of the care of the patient. The essay written by
Francis W. Peabody is an inspiring call to all physicians to remember that the care of a patient must be
completely personal. "The clinical picture is not just a
photograph of a man sick in bed; it is an impressionistic painting of the patient in his home, his work, his
relations, his friends, his joys, sorrow, hopes, and
fears."

The physician, no matter how knowledgeable or
skillful, will invariably encounter problems which are
not amenable to definitive treatment. As physicians we
tend to view the patient who responds to our treatment
as a triumph and the dying patient as a failure. This
perception is erroneous and may cause the physician to
withdraw from this patient whenever he feels he has no
specific therapy to contribute. The continuing care and
interest of the physician can be the most sustaining
pillar of support for the terminal patient and his family. James Bigelow, M.D., described a physician's
duties in the following order, "to diagnose, to initiate

treatment, to offer relief of symptoms, and to provide safe passage. A safe passage implies a mutual confidence and trust between patient and physician that allows the sick to feel that all that could be done to save had been done, and the anxiety would be diminished, even unto death."

We draw attention to the attitude of society in general and physicians in particular towards persons with progressive or terminal illness, dementia, and mental illness and the ways in which the lot of these patients can be improved. Several essays in this book are devoted to the role of the physician in the face of incurable illness in a patient or colleague. Other essays provide practical guidelines for the physician who must help patients deal with acute grief, chronic physical debility, intractable pain, and terminal illness. We have also included contributions on cancer and mental retardation as seen from the perspective of the patient and his family. Among the most awesome responsibilities of the physician is the comforting of the patient and his family in a setting where scientific knowledge is of little avail. We wish to raise the consciousness of physicians that technologic advances do not render obsolete the need to express care and compassion. This book is dedicated to humanism which is integral to the practice of medicine.

THE CARE OF THE PATIENT

Francis W. Peabody

It is probably fortunate that most systems of education are constantly under the fire of general criticism, for if education were left solely in the hands of teachers the chances are good that it would soon deteriorate. Medical education, however, is less likely to suffer from such stagnation, for whenever the lay public stops criticizing the type of modern doctor, the medical profession itself may be counted on to stir up the stagnant pool and cleanse it of its sedimentary deposit. The most common criticism made at present by older practitioners is that young graduates have been taught a great deal about the mechanism of disease, but very little about the practice of medicine—or, to put it more bluntly, they are too "scientific" and do not know how to take care of patients.

One is, of course, somewhat tempted to question how completely fitted for his life-work the practitioner of the older generation was when he first entered on it, and

1

how much the haze of time has led him to confuse what he learned in the school of medicine with what he acquired in the harder school of experience. But the indictment is a serious one and it is concurred in by numerous recent graduates, who find that in the actual practice of medicine they encounter many situations which they had not been led to anticipate and which they are not prepared to meet effectively. Where there is so much smoke there is undoubtedly a good deal of fire, and the problem for teachers and for students is to consider what they can do to extinguish whatever is left of this smoldering distrust.

To begin with, the fact must be accepted that one cannot expect to become a skillful practitioner of medicine in the four or five years allotted to the medical curriculum. Medicine is not a trade to be learned but a profession to be entered. It is an ever-widening field that requires continued study and prolonged experience in close contact with the sick. All that the medical school can hope to do is to supply the foundations on which to build. When one considers the amazing progress of science in its relation to medicine during the last thirty years, and the enormous mass of scientific material which must be made available to the modern physician, it is not surprising that the schools have tended to concern themselves more and more with this phase of the educational problem. And while they have been absorbed in the difficult task of digesting and correlating new knowledge, it has been easy to overlook the fact that the application of the principles of science to the diagnosis and treatment of disease is only one limited aspect of medical practice. The practice of medicine in its broadest sense includes the whole relationship of the physician with his patient. It is an art, based to an increasing extent on the medical sciences, but comprising much that still remains outside the realm of any science. The art of medicine and the science of medicine are not antagonistic but supplementary to each other. There is no more contradiction between the science of medicine and the art of medicine than between the science of aeronautics and the art of flying. Good practice presupposes an understanding of the sciences which contribute to the structure of modern medicine, but it is obvious that sound professional training would include a much broader equipment.

The problem that I wish to consider, therefore, is whether this larger view of the profession cannot be approached even under the conditions imposed by the present curriculum of a medical school. Can the practitioner's art be grafted on the main trunk of the fundamental sciences in such a way that there may arise a symmetrical growth, like an expanding tree, the leaves of which shall be for the "healing of the nations"?

The physician who speaks of the care of patients is naturally thinking about circumstances as they exist in the practice of medicine; but the teacher who is attempting to train medical students is immediately confronted by the fact that, even if he would, he cannot make the conditions under which he has to teach clinical medicine exactly similar to those of actual practice.

The primary difficulty is that instruction has to be carried out largely in the wards and dispensaries of hospitals rather than in the patient's home and the physician's office. Now the essence of the practice of medicine is that it is an intensely personal matter, and one of the chief differences between private practice and hospital practice is that the latter always tends to become impersonal. At first sight this may not appear to be a very vital point, but it is, as a matter of fact, the crux of the whole situation. The treatment of a disease may be entirely impersonal; the care of a patient must be completely personal. The significance of the intimate personal relationship between physician and patient cannot be too strongly emphasized, for in an extraordinarily large number of cases both diagnosis and treatment are directly dependent on it, and the failure of the young physician to establish this relationship accounts for much of his ineffectiveness in the care of patients.

Hospitals—like other institutions founded with the highest human ideals—are apt to deteriorate into dehumanized machines, and even the physician who has the patient's welfare most at heart finds that pressure of work forces him to give most of his attention to the critically sick and to whose diseases are a menace to the public health. In such cases he must first treat the specific disease, and there then remains little time in which to cultivate more than a superficial personal contact with the patients. Moreover, the circumstances under which the physician sees the patient are not wholly favorable to the establishment of the intimate personal relationship that exists in private practice, for one of the outstanding features of hospitalization is that it completely removes the patient from his accustomed environment. This may, of course, be entirely desirable, and one of the main reasons for sending a person into the hospital is to get him away from home surroundings which, be he rich or poor, are often unfavorable to recovery; but at the same time it is equally important for the physician to know the exact character of those surroundings.

Everybody, sick or well, is affected in one way or another, consciously or subconsciously, by the material and spiritual forces that bear on his life, and especially to the sick such forces may act as powerful stimulants or depressants. When the general practitioner goes into the home of a patient, he may know the whole background of the family life from past experience; but even when he comes as a stranger he has every opportunity to find out what manner of man his patient is, and what kind of circumstances makes his life. He gets a hint of financial anxiety or of domestic incompatibility; he may find himself confronted by a querulous, exacting, self-centered patient, or by a gentle invalid overawed by a dominating family; and as he appreciates how these circumstances are reacting on the patient he dispenses sympathy, encouragement, or discipline. What is spoken of as a "clinical picture" is not just a photograph of a man sick in bed; it is an impressionistic painting of the patient surrounded by his home, his work, his relations, his friends, his joys, sorrows, hopes, and fears. Now, all of this background of sickness which bears so strongly on the symptomatology is liable to be lost sight of in the hospital: I say "liable to" because it is not by any means always lost sight of, and because I believe that by making a constant and conscious effort one can almost always bring it out into its proper perspective. The difficulty is that in the hospital one gets into the habit of using the oil immersion lens instead of the low power, and focuses too intently on the center of the field.

When a patient enters a hospital, the first thing that commonly happens to him is that he loses his personal identity. He is generally referred to, not as Henry Jones, but as "that case of mitral stenosis in the second bed on the left." There are plenty of reasons why this is so, and the point is, in itself, relatively unimportant; but the trouble is that it leads, more or less directly, to the patient being treated as a case of mitral stenosis, and not as a sick man. The disease is treated, but Henry

Jones, lying awake nights while he worries about his wife and children, represents a problem that is much more complex than the pathologic physiology of mitral stenosis, and he is apt to improve very slowly unless a discerning intern discovers why it is that even large doses of digitalis fail to slow his heart rate. Henry happens to have heart disease, but he is not disturbed so much by dyspnea as he is by anxiety of the future, and a talk with an understanding physician who tries to make the situation clear to him, and then gets the social service worker to find a suitable occupation, does more to straighten him out than a book full of drugs and diets. Henry has an excellent example of a certain type of heart disease, and he is glad that all the staff find him interesting, for it makes him feel that they will do the best they can to cure him; but just because he is an interesting case he does not cease to be a human being with very human hopes and fears. Sickness produces an abnormally sensitive emotional state in almost everyone, and in many cases the emotional state repercusses, as it were, on the organic disease. The pneumonia would probably run its course in a week, regardless of treatment, but the experienced physician knows that by quieting the cough, getting the patient to sleep, and giving a bit of encouragement, he can save his patient's strength and lift him through many distressing hours. The institutional eye tends to become focused on the lung, and it forgets that the lung is only one member of the body.

But if teachers and students are inclined to take a limited point of view even toward interesting cases of organic disease, they fall into more serious error in their attitude toward a large group of patients who do not show objective, organic, pathologic conditions and who are generally spoken of as having "nothing the matter with them." Up to a certain point, as long as they are regarded as diagnostic problems, they command attention; but as soon as the physician has assured himself that they do not have organic disease, he passes them over lightly.

Take the case of a young woman, for instance, who entered the hospital with a history of nausea and discomfort in the upper part of the abdomen after eating. Mrs. Brown had "suffered many things of many physicians." Each of them gave her a tonic and limited her diet. She stopped eating everything that any of her physicians advised her to omit, and is now living on a little milk with a few crackers; but her symptoms persist. The history suggests a possible gastric ulcer or gall-stones, and with a proper desire to study the case thoroughly, she is given a test meal, gastric analysis, and duodenal intubation, and roentgen-ray examinations are made of the gastro-intestinal tract and gall-bladder. All of these diagnostic methods give negative results: that is, they do not show evidence of any structural change. The case immediately becomes much less interesting than if it had turned out to be a gastric ulcer with atypical symptoms. The visiting physician walks by and says, "Well, there's nothing the matter with her." The clinical clerk says, "I did an awful lot of work on that case and it turned out to be nothing at all." The intern, who wants to clear out the ward to make room for some interesting cases, says, "Mrs. Brown, you can send for your clothes and go home tomorrow. There is really nothing the matter with you, and fortunately you have not got any of the serious troubles we suspected. We have used all the most modern and scientific methods and we find that there is no reason why you should not eat anything you want to. I'll give you a tonic to take when you go home." Same story, same colored medicine! Mrs. Brown goes home, somewhat better for the rest in new surroundings, thinking that nurses are kind and physicians are pleasant, but that they do not seem to know much about the sort of medicine that will touch her trouble. She takes up her life and the symptoms return—and then she tries chiropractic, or perhaps Christian Science.

It is rather fashionable to say the modern physician has become "too scientific." Now, was it too scientific, with all the stomach tubes and blood counts and roentgen-ray examinations? Not at all. Mrs. Brown's symptoms might have been due to a gastric ulcer or to gall-stones, and after such a long course it was only proper to use every method that might help to clear the diagnosis. Was it, perhaps, not scientific enough? The popular conception of a scientist is a man who works in a laboratory and who uses instruments of precision is as inaccurate as it is superficial, for a scientist is known, not by his technical processes but by his intellectual processes; and the essence of the scientific method of thought is that it proceeds in an orderly manner toward the establishment of a truth. Now the chief criticism to be made of the way Mrs. Brown's case was handled is that the staff was contented with a half-truth. The investigation of the patient was decidedly unscientific in that it stopped short of even an attempt to determine the real cause of the symptoms. As soon as organic disease could be excluded the whole problem was given up, but the symptoms persisted. Speaking candidly, the case was a medical failure in spite of the fact that the patient went home with the assurance that there was "nothing the matter" with her.

A good many "Mrs. Browns," male and female, come to hospitals, and a great many more go to private physicians. They are all characterized by the presence of symptoms that cannot be accounted for by organic disease, and they are all liable to be told that they have "nothing the matter" with them. Now, my own experience as a hospital physician has been rather long and varied, and I have always found that, from my point of view, hospitals are particularly interesting and cheerful places; but I am fairly certain that, except for a few low-grade morons and some poor wretches who want to get in out of the cold, there are not many people who become hospital patients unless there is something the matter with them. And, by the same token, I doubt whether there are many people, except those stupid creatures who would rather go to the physician than go to the theater, who spend their money on visiting private physicians unless there is something the matter with them. In hospital and in private practice, however, one finds this same type of patient, and many physicians whom I have questioned agree in saying that, excluding cases of acute infection, approximately half of their patients complained of symptoms for which an adequate organic cause could not be discovered. Numerically, then, these patients constitute a large group and their fees go a long way toward spreading butter on the doctor's bread. Medically speaking, they are not serious cases as regards prospective death, but they are often extremely serious as regards prospective life. Their symptoms will rarely prove fatal, but their lives will be long and miserable, and they may end by nearly exhausting their families and friends. Death is not the worst thing in the world, and to help a man to a happy and useful career may be more of a service than the saving of life.

What is the matter with all these patients? Technically, most of them come under the broad heading of the "psychoneuroses"; but for practical purposes many of them may be regarded as patients whose subjective symptoms are due to disturbances of the physiologic activity of one or more organs or systems. These symptoms may depend on an increase or a decrease of a normal function, or an abnormality of function, or merely on the subjects becoming conscious of a wholly normal function that normally goes on unnoticed; and this last conception indicates that there is a close relationship between the appearance of the symptoms and the threshold of the patient's nervous reactions. The ultimate causes of these disturbances are to be found, not in any gross structural changes of the organism involved, but rather in nervous influences emanating from the emotional or intellectual life which, directly or indirectly, affect in one way or another organs that are under either voluntary or involuntary control.

All of you have had experiences that have brought home the way in which emotional reactions affect organic functions. Some of you have been nauseated while anxiously waiting for an important examination to begin, and a few may even have vomited; others have been seized by an attack of diarrhea under the same circumstances. Some of you have polyuria before making a speech, and others have felt thumping extrasystoles or a pounding tachycardia before a football game. Some of you have noticed rapid, shallow breathing when listening to a piece of bad news, and others know the type of occipital headache, with pain down the muscles of the back of the neck, that comes from nervous anxiety and fatigue.

These are all simple examples of the way that emotional reactions may upset the normal functioning of an organ. Vomiting and diarrhea are due to abnormalities of the motor function of the gastro-intestinal tract—one to the production of an active reversed peristalsis of the stomach and a relaxation of the cardiac sphincter, the other to hyperperistalsis of the large intestine. The polyuria is caused by vasomotor changes in renal circulation, similar in character to the vasomotor changes that take place in the peripheral vessels in blushing and blanching of the skin, and in addition there are quite possibly associated changes in the rate of blood flow and in blood pressure. Tachycardia and extrasystoles indicate that not only the rate but also the rhythm of the heart is under a nervous control that can be demonstrated in the intact human being as well as in the experimental animal. The ventilatory function of the respiration is extraordinarily subject to nervous influences; so much so, in fact, that the study of the respiration in man is associated with peculiar difficulties. Rate, depth, and rhythm of breathing are easily upset by even minor stimuli, and in extreme cases the disturbance in total ventilation is sometimes so great that gaseous exchange becomes affected. Thus, I remember an emotional young woman who developed a respiratory neurosis with deep and rapid breathing, and expired so much carbon dioxide that the symptoms of tetany ensued. The explanation of the occipital headaches and of so many pains in the muscles of the back is not entirely clear, but they appear to be associated with changes in muscular tone or with prolonged states of contraction. There is certainly a very intimate correlation between mental tenseness and muscular tenseness, and whatever methods are used to produce mental relaxation will usually cause muscular relaxation, together with relief of this type of pain. A similar condition is found in so-called writers' cramp, in which the painful muscles of the hand result; not from manual work, but from mental work.

One might go much further, but these few illustrations will suffice to recall the infinite number of ways in which physiologic functions may be upset by emotional stimuli, and the manner in which the resulting disturbances of function manifest themselves as symptoms. These symptoms, although obviously not due to anatomic changes, may, nevertheless, be very disturbing and distressing, and there is nothing imaginary about them. Emotional vomiting is just as real as the vomiting due to pyloric obstruction, and so-called "nervous headaches" may be as painful as if they were due to a brain tumor. Moreover, it must be remembered that symptoms based on functional disturbances may be present in a patient who has, at the same time, organic disease, and in such cases the determination of the causes of the different symptoms may be an extremely difficult matter. Every one accepts the relationship between the common functional symptoms and nervous reactions, for convincing evidence is to be found in the fact that under ordinary circumstances the symptoms disappear just as soon as the emotional cause has passed. But what happens if the cause does not pass away? What if, instead of having to face a single three-hour examination, one has to face a life of being constantly on the rack? The emotional stimulus persists, and continues to produce the disturbances of function. As with all nervous reactions the longer the process goes on, or the more frequently it goes on, the easier it is for it to go on. The unusual nervous track becomes an established path. After a time, the symptom and the subjective discomfort that it produces come to occupy the center of the picture, and the causative factors recede into a hazy background. The patient no longer thinks, "I cannot stand this life," but he says out loud, "I cannot stand this nausea and vomiting. I must go to see a stomach specialist."

Quite possibly your comment on this will be that the symptoms of such "neurotic" patients are well known, and they ought to go to a neurologist or a psychiatrist and not to an internist or a general practitioner. In an era of internal medicine, however, which takes pride in the fact that it concerns itself with the functional capacity of organs rather than with mere structural changes, and which has developed so many "functional tests" of kidneys, heart, and liver, is it not rather narrow-minded to limit one's interest to those disturbances of function which are based on anatomic abnormalities? There are other reasons, too, why most of these "functional" cases belong to the field of general medicine. In the first place, the differential diagnosis between organic disease and pure functional disturbance is often extremely difficult, and it needs the broad training in the use of general clinical and laboratory methods which forms the equipment of the internist. Diagnosis is the first step in treatment. In the second place, the patients themselves frequently prefer to go to a medical practitioner rather than to a psychiatrist, and in the long run it is probably better for them to get straightened out without having what they often consider the stigma of having been "nervous" cases. A limited number, it is true, are so refractory or so complex that the aid of the psychiatrist must be sought, but the majority can be helped by the internist without highly specialized psychologic technic, if the medical practitioner will appreciate the significance of functional disturbances and interest himself in their treatment. The physician who does take these cases seriously—one might say scientifically—has the great satisfaction of seeing some of his patients get well, not as the result of drugs or as the result of the disease having run its course, but as the result of his own individual efforts.

Here, then, is a great group of patients in which it is not disease but the man or the woman who needs to be treated. In general practice physicians are so busy with the critically sick, and in clinical teaching they are so concerned with training students in physical diagnosis and attempting to show them all types of organic disease, that they do not pay as much attention as they should to the functional disorders. Many a student enters upon his career having hardly heard of them except in his course in psychiatry, and without the faintest conception of how large a part they will play in his future practice. At best, his method of treatment is apt to be a cheerful reassurance combined with a placebo. The successful diagnosis and treatment of these patients, however, depends almost wholly in the establishment of that intimate personal contact between physician and patient which forms the basis of private practice. Without this, it is quite impossible for the physician to get an idea of the problems and troubles that lie behind so many functional disorders. If students are to obtain any insight into this field of medicine, they must also be given opportunities to build up the same type of personal relationship with their patients.

Is there, then, anything inherent in the conditions of clinical teaching in a general hospital that makes this impossible? Can you form a personal relationship in an impersonal institution? Can you accept the fact that your patient is entirely removed from his natural environment and then reconstruct the backgound of environment from the history, from the family, from a visit to the home or workshop, and from the information obtained by the social-service worker? And while you are building up this environmental background, can you enter into the same personal relationship that you ought to have in private practice? If you can do all this, and I know form experience that you can, then the study of medicine in the hospital actually becomes the practice of medicine, and the treatment of disease immediately takes its proper place in the larger problem of the care of the patient.

When a patient goes to a physician he usually has confidence that the physician is the best, or at least the best available, person to help him in what is, for the time being, his most important trouble. He relies on him as on a sympathetic advisor and a wise professional counsellor. When a patient goes to a hospital he has confidence in the reputation of the institution, but, it is hardly necessary to add that he also hopes to come into contact with some individual who personifies the institution and will also take a human interest in him. It is obvious that the first physician to see the patient is in this strategic position—and in hospitals all students can have the satisfaction of being regarded as physicians.

Here, for instance, is a poor fellow who has just been jolted to the hospital in an ambulance. A string of questions about himself and his family has been fired at him, his valuables and even his clothes have been taken away from him, and he is wheeled into the ward on a truck, miserable, scared, defenseless, and, in his nakedness, unable to run away. He is lifted into a bed, becomes conscious of the fact that he is the center of interest in the ward, wishes that he had stayed at home among friends, and, just as he is beginning to take stock of his surroundings, finds that a thermometer is being stuck under his tongue. It is all strange and new, and he wonders what is going to happen next. The next thing that does happen is that a man in a long white coat sits down by his bedside, and starts to talk to him.

Now it happens that according to our system of clinical instruction that man is usually a medical student. Do you see what an opportunity you have? The foundation of your whole relation with that patient is laid in those first few minutes of contact, just as happens in private practice. Here is a worried, lonely, suffering man, and if you begin by approaching him with sympathy, tact, and consideration, you get his confidence and he becomes *your* patient. Interns and visiting physicians may come and go, and the hierarchy gives them precedence; but if you make the most of your opportunities he will regard you as his personal physician, and all the rest as mere consultants. Of course, you must not drop him after you have taken the history and made your physical examination. Once your relationship with him has been established, you must foster it by every means. Watch his condition closely and he will see that you are alert professionally. Make time to have little talks with him—and these talks need not always be about his symptoms. Remember that you want to know him as a man, and this means you must know about his family and friends, his work and his play. What kind of person is he—cheerful, depressed, introspective, careless, conscientious, mentally keen or dull? Look out for all the little incidental things that you can do for his comfort. These, too, are a part of "the care of the patient." Some of them will fall technically into the field of "nursing," but you will always be profoundly grateful for any nursing technique that you have acquired. It is worth your while to get the nurse to teach you the right way to feed a patient, change the bed, or give a bed pan. Do you know the practical tricks that make a dyspneic patient comfortable? Assume some responsibility for these apparently minor points and you will find that it is when you are doing some such friendly service, rather than when you are a formal questioner, that the patient suddenly starts to unburden himself, and a flood of light is thrown on the situation.

Meantime, of course, you will have been active along strictly medical lines, and by the time your clinical and laboratory examinations are completed you will be surprised to see how intimately you know your patient, not only as an interesting case but also as a sick human being. And everything you have picked up about him will be of value in the subsequent handling of the situation. Suppose, for instance you find conclusive evidence that his symptoms are due to organic disease: say, to a gastric ulcer. As soon as you face the problem of laying out his regimen you find that it is one thing to write an examination paper on the treatment of gastric ulcer and quite another thing to treat John Smith, who happens to have a gastic ulcer. You want to begin by giving him rest in bed and a special diet for eight weeks. Rest means both nervous and physical rest. Can he get it best at home or in the hospital? What are the conditions at home? If you keep him in the hospital, it is probably good for him to see certain people, and bad for him to see others. He has business problems that must be considered. What kind of compromise can you make on them? How about the financial implications of eight weeks in bed followed by a period of convalescence? Is it, on the whole, wiser to try a strict regimen for a shorter period, and, if he does not improve, take up the question of operation sooner than is in general advisable? These and many similar problems arise in the course of the treatment of almost every patient, and they have to be looked at, not from the abstact point of view of the treatment of the disease, but from the concrete point of view of the care of the individual.

Suppose, on the other hand, that all your clinical and

laboratory examinations turn out entirely negative as far as revealing any evidence of organic disease is concerned. Then you are in the difficult position of not having discovered the explanation of the patient's symptoms. You have merely assured yourself that certain conditions are not present. Of course, the first thing you have to consider is whether these symptoms are the result of organic disease in such an early stage that you cannot definitely recognize it. This problem is often extremely perplexing, requiring great clinical experience for its solution, and often you will be forced to fall back on time in which to watch developments. If, however, you finally exclude recognizable organic disease, and the probability of early or very slight organic disease, it becomes necessary to consider whether the symptomatology may be due to a functional disorder which is caused by nervous or emotional influences. You know a good deal about the personal life of your patient by this time, but perhaps there is nothing that stands out as an obvious etiologic factor, and it becomes necessary to sit down for a long, intimate talk with him to discover what has remained hidden.

Sometimes it is well to explain to the patient, by obvious examples, how it is that emotional states may bring about symptoms similar to his own, so that he will understand what you are driving at and will cooperate with you. Often the best way is to go back to the very beginning and try to find out the circumstances of the patient's life at the time the symptoms first began. The association between symptoms and cause may have been simpler and more direct at the onset, at least in the patient's mind, for as time goes on, and the symptoms become more pronounced and distressing, there is a natural tendency for the symptoms to occupy so much of the foreground of the picture that the background is completely obliterated. Sorrow, disappointment, anxiety, self-distrust, thwarted ideals or ambitions in social, business, or personal life, and particularly what are called maladaptations to these conditions—these are among the commonest and simplest factors that initiate and perpetuate the functional disturbances. Perhaps you will find that the digestive disturbances began at the time the patient was in serious financial difficulties, and that they have recurred whenever he is worried about money matters. Or you may find that ten years ago a physician told the patient he had heart disease, cautioning him "not to worry about it." For ten years the patient has never mentioned the subject, but he has avoided every exertion, and has lived with the idea that sudden death was in store for him. You will find that physicians, by wrong diagnosis and ill-considered statements, are responsible for many a wrecked life, and you will discover that it is much easier to make a wrong diagnosis than it is to unmake it. Or, again, you may find that the pain in this woman's back made its appearance when she first felt her domestic unhappiness, and that this man's headaches have been associated, not with long hours of work, but with a constant depression due to unfulfilled ambitions. The causes are manifold and the manifestations protean. Sometimes the mechanism of cause and effect is obvious; sometimes it becomes apparent only after a very tangled skein has been unraveled.

If the establishment of an intimate personal relationship is necessary in the diagnosis of functional disturbances, it becomes doubly necessary in their treatment. Unless there is complete confidence in the sympathetic understanding of the physician as well as in his professional skill, very little can be accomplished; but granted that you have been able to get close enough to the patient to discover the cause of the trouble, you will find that a general hospital is not at all an impossible place for the treatment of functional disturbances. The hospital has, indeed, the advantage that the entire reputation of the institution and all that it represents in the way of facilities for diagnosis and treatment go to enhance the confidence which the patient has in the individual physician who represents it. This gives the very young physician a hold on his patients that he could scarcely hope to have without its support. Another advantage is that hospital patients are removed from their usual environment, for the treatment of functional disturbances is often easier when patients are away from friends, relatives, home, work, and, indeed, everything that is associated with their daily life. It is true that in a public ward one cannot obtain complete isolation in the sense that this is a part of the Weir Mitchell treatment, but the main object is accomplished if one has obtained the psychologic effect of isolation which comes with an entirely new and unaccustomed atmosphere. The conditions, therefore, under which you as students, come into contact with patients with functional disturbances are not wholly unfavorable, and with very little effort they can be made to simulate closely the conditions in private practice.

It is not my purpose, however, to go into a discussion of the methods of treating functional disturbances, and I have dwelt on the subject only because these cases illustrate so clearly the vital importance of the personal relationship between physician and patient in the practice of medicine. In all your patients whose symptoms are of functional origin, the whole problem of diagnosis and treatment depends on your insight into the patient's character and personal life, and in every case of organic disease there are complex interactions between the pathologic processes and the intellectual processes which you must appreciate and consider if you would be a wise clinician. There are moments, of course, in cases of serious illness when you will think solely of the disease and its treatment; but when the corner is turned and the immediate crisis is passed, you must give your attention to the patient. Disease in man is never exactly the same as disease in an experimental animal, for in man the disease at once affects and is affected by what we call the emotional life. Thus, the physician who attempts to take care of a patient while he neglects this factor is as unscientific as the investigator who neglects to control all the conditions that may affect his experiment. The good physician knows his patients through and through, and his knowledge is bought dearly. Time, sympathy, and understanding must be lavishly dispensed, but the reward is to be found in that personal bond which forms the greatest satisfaction of the practice of medicine. One of the essential qualities of the clinician is interest in humanity, for the secret of the care of the patient is in caring for the patient.

THE CARE OF THE PATIENT: FRANCIS PEABODY REVISITED

Pauline L. Rabin
and David Rabin

This classic essay with its fabric of pristine humanism, its universality, and its timelessness embodies the noblest aspirations of the medical profession. Peabody gave this address at the Harvard Medical School during a course on the care of the patient. Dr. Joseph Pratt was in the audience and subsequently wrote: "After the lecture I talked with Dr. Peabody. His address doubtless made a deep impression on the audience but there was no evidence of unusual approval. In a few minutes the hall was emptied and we were alone."[1] Since that day in 1926, Peabody's words have become a paradigm for all physicians.

His talk covered three chief topics. The first is devoted to the importance of individualizing medical care. Long before the introduction of the SMAC 46 battery to which so many patients are subjected even before they see their physician, Peabody cautioned the medical profession in the following words: "The essence of the practice of medicine is that it is an intensely personal matter. The treatment of a disease may be entirely impersonal; the care of a patient must be completely personal. The significance of the intimate personal relationship between physician and patient cannot be too strongly emphasized, for in an extraordinarily large number of cases both diagnosis and treatment are directly dependent on it." This philosophy was already deeply ingrained in Peabody while still a medical student. In 1906, addressing the Boylston Medical Society on the treatment of diabetes, he said: "We must not forget in treating diabetes that we are treating a man and not a disease."[2]

The following example bears out Peabody's message. A patient with cancer of the breast had great confidence in her oncologist. She was, however, concerned about metastases and was becoming increasingly depressed. Whenever she asked him a question about her illness he would give her an answer based on statistical results from the literature. The patient inferred from this that to him she was no more than an impersonal dot in a computer print-out. Clearly, statistical information is extremely valuable. The physician, however, should not hide behind numbers to avoid dealing with the patient's underlying anxiety which prompted those questions.

His second concern is a call to awareness about the dehumanizing experience which so often accompanies hospitalization. Peabody displays remarkable insight of the forces which tend to depersonalize the patient who enters a hospital. He emphasizes the difficulties of getting to know the patient as an individual in a hospital setting. These features have been magnified over the past fifty years. As soon as a patient is registered in a medical center today, his entire past record and laboratory data can be obtained by punching the correct code into a computer. This, of course, provides invaluable information. The various teams of consultants and even the patient's personal physician and resident may become so absorbed in receiving the computerized information that they may spend less time with the patient. These realities can be overcome by adherence to Peabody's credo. "What is spoken of as a 'clinical picture' is not just a photograph of a man sick in bed; it is an impressionistic painting of the patient surrounded by his home, his work, his relations, his friends, his joys, sorrows, hopes, and fears. This all bears so strongly on the symptomatology and is liable to be lost sight of in the hospital." These concerns apply equally to current private practice. Peabody was the great champion of the general practitioner who knew the patient and his family intimately. Today house calls are virtually obsolete and patients may be seen by a succession of specialists, none of whom have a clear picture or understanding of the man or woman who is their patient.

His third topic deals with the care of patients who have symptoms for which an organic cause cannot be determined. Peabody devotes a considerable segment of his essay towards improving the attitude of physicians to those patients who do not show objective, organic, pathologic conditions, and who are generally spoken of as having "nothing the matter with them." Peabody thought that this group of patients constituted up to half of any physician's practice, and this is probably true today. It is known that the majority of antidepressants and minor tranquilizers are prescribed by non-psychiatrists. Peabody advocates an approach which includes a thorough knowledge of psychological factors operative in the patient's life. This can only be obtained by spending time with the person and gaining his confidence about intimate personal history. Rather than communicating to the patient that there is "nothing the matter," one should take the time to explain "how it is that emotional states may bring about symptoms similar to his own." It has been well documented that education of patients about their illness and about psychological issues is an inherent and critical part of all medical treatment. Today, this approach is appreciated as an important adjuvant in the care of the patient, especially those patients with chronic diseases.

When we initially read this paper, we were inspired by the clinical sensitivity linked with scientific perspective but were surprised by an omission of a discussion on the role of the physician with terminally ill and dying patients. Jacob Bigelow, addressing a group of medical students in 1858, had described the duties of a physician to encompass diagnosis, treatment, the relief of symptoms, and the provision of safe passage.[3] By safe passage is meant the support and ready availability of the physician to his or her patient until death. Although Peabody did not actually discuss the terminally ill in his famous address, he was communicating another very important message regarding this subject to his audience by his very presence there. It was known that he was at that time suffering from an inoperable cancer. Yet, he continued to function, teach, and care for his patients as long as he was able. Thus, he was an example of how a person can accept illness and live alongside it with dignity and purpose. Although the quantity of life granted to him was short (he died at the age of forty-seven), the quality of his life was enriched by his dedication to his work, his devotion to his family, and the support he received from his friends. Langdon Warner, a lifelong friend, was moved to write his account of those remarkable visits. "You came hesitating, perhaps, and wondering how you could stand it. But you smoked, gossiped, and reported the news; discussed a marriage, birth, or a death; told your troubles, took some of the invalid's grapes, and left. There had been no sad-eyed bravery about it, no attempt to ignore the obvious. And all this time when our hearts were standing still with the pity of it, his task was gently to show us that there was no need for horror."[4]

There have been dramatic changes in medicine in the fifty years since Peabody died. Much would have delighted and perhaps even amazed him. We suspect, however, that he would have viewed some of the changes with deep apprehension. The cost of medical care now approaches 300 billion dollars annually or 10.5% of the GNP, and despite this staggering figure, good medical care is not readily available to all citizens.[5] In 1923 he wrote, "The primary function of a municipal hospital is without question, to provide the best care for the sick poor of the city.... The municipal hospital must be prepared at all times to admit any and every citizen genuinely in need of medical aid.... In a municipal institution, even more than in a private institution, there is need for trained social workers. The duty of the city towards the health of its citizens certainly extends beyond the walls of the hospital."[6] Today, the care of the poor and those without adequate medical insurance is delegated to the already overburdened general hospitals which are supported by increasingly depleted municipal funds. Some city hospitals have in fact been forced to close. The health plight of the poor is becoming critical.

How would this man who chose Boston City Hospital over choice appointments at Johns Hopkins, Yale, and Stanford have viewed the burgeoning hospital for profit phenomenon? How would this man who spent the last days of his life completing an essay on the soul of the clinic have reacted to the marketing of health care by enormous corporations?[7] He would surely have been exercised by the growing medical needs of the chronically ill, the aged and by a nursing home population of 1.3 million which is expected to climb to 2 million within a decade. Nor would he have avoided confronting the awesome ethical dilemmas that face physicians engaged in the care of chronic, debilitated patients in nursing homes.[8]

In all probability, he would have shared Lewis Thomas's concern about the widening gap between the physician and his patient and might well have commended Lewis Thomas's turn of phrase "Medicine is no longer the laying on of hands, it is more like the reading of signals from machines."[9] He would certainly have agreed also with Thomas's concern for the changing nature of the medical profession today. Writes Thomas, "If I were a medical student or an intern, just getting ready to begin, I would be apprehensive that my real job, caring for sick people, might soon be taken away, leaving me with the quite different occupation of looking after machines." Peabody's scientific contributions were outstanding. Had he lived another few years it is very possible that he would have shared with his friend Minot the Nobel prize for the discovery of liver therapy for pernicious anemia. Nonetheless, his legacy to medicine is eternal. He was the compleat physician, clinical scientist, teacher, healer, counselor, confidant, and friend to his patients.

References

1. Pratt, J.H. The personality of the physician. *N. Engl. J. Med.* 1936; 214:364-370.

2. Boylston Medical Society Records, 1899-1908 (bound volume in Harvard Medical School Library), pp. 307-308.

3. Krant, J. *Dying and Dignity.* Springfield, Illinois; Charles C. Thomas, 1974, p. 60. A somewhat different quotation is found in Bigelow, J. *Brief Exposition of Rationale Medicine.* Boston; Phillips, Sampson and Company, 1858.

4. Warner, L. Quoted in *Francis Weld Peabody, 1881-1927, a Memoir.* Privately printed (by Francis G. Peabody), Riverside Press, Cambridge, 1933, pp. 69-70.

5. Starr, P. The laissez-faire elixir. *The New Republic* 1983; 561:19-23.

6. Peabody, F.W. The function of a municipal hospital. *The Boston Medical and Surgical Journal* 1923; 189:125-129.

7. Peabody, F.W. The soul of the clinic. J.A.M.A. 1928; 90:1193-1197.

8. Hilfiker, D. Allowing the debilitated to die. *N. Engl. J. Med.* 1983; 308:716-719.

9. Thomas, L. *The Youngest Science.* New York; The Viking Press, 1983.

COMPOUNDING THE ORDEAL OF ALS:
Isolation from My Fellow Physicians

David Rabin, Pauline L. Rabin, and Roni C. Rabin

It has been three years since my first symptoms suggested a diagnosis of amyotrophic lateral sclerosis
(ALS). The pain and anguish of this illness are known
to most physicians and are an inevitable accompani-
ment of the disease, but there are other unpleasant
aspects that are avoidable. In this article I want to
relate my personal story and to emphasize the extra-
ordinary change that my illness brought about in my
interrelations with fellow physicians.

I turned forty-five in January 1979. I was then director of endocrinology at the Vanderbilt Medical Center,
and my research in the areas of metabolism and reproduction was flourishing. I was supremely happy with
my wife and family; we traveled often and enjoyed an
active and varied social life. My wife and I had both

graduated from the University of Witwatersrand in Johannesburg, South Africa. After completing our postgraduate education at Johns Hopkins Medical Center, we had stayed on the faculty there for nearly a decade. We then spent five years in Israel working at the Hadassah Medical Center, and in 1975 we returned to the States and settled in Nashville.

My years at Vanderbilt have been very happy. The foundation for this happiness is the atmosphere of unusual cordiality and collegiality that is the hallmark of this medical school. I had known the rampant political intrigues of the academic world and had found them abhorrent, but at Vanderbilt there is a spirit of cooperation and collaboration that makes going to work a pleasure. Politics always exist in an intellectual and competitive environment. What is unique about Vanderbilt is the choice it offers to eschew such distractions and concentrate on the fundamentals of one's profession. As a result, my years here have been characterized by academic advancement, many friendships, and a sense of acceptance by students, house staff, and colleagues. This background is important to the story I am about to relate because, whereas I had previously been "at" Hopkins and "at" Hadassah, I now felt I was "of" Vanderbilt.

During my early years at medical school I had steeped myself in the study of neurologic anatomy and had shown precocious talent in clinical neurology. I did not choose neurology, however. My reasons were clear: the diagnostic problem seemed largely an academic exercise—so little, if anything, could be done for the patient in a definitive therapeutic way. The years, as well as my own illness, however, have taught me how wrong it is to focus on definitive therapy and how much can and should be done for the patient, even when one is confronted with so-called incurable illness. In any event, although my field became endocrinology, my knowledge of neurology did not evaporate. How ironic this would turn out to be. In June of 1979 I noticed some stiffness in my legs. Within two short weeks I discovered quite by chance that my reflexes had become pathologically brisk. When I could no longer dismiss fasciculation as mere "restless legs" and it became clear that there were no sensory symptoms, the diagnosis of ALS reached my consciousness despite every attempt at denial.

This story will confine itself to the effects of my illness on my relationships with my fellow physicians—whether they were my personal physicians, professional colleagues, or old friends. My strategy was to avoid disclosure of my illness for as long as possible, for the following reasons. First of all, my wife and I agreed that ignorance was a blessing, especially for our children, who would eventually have to endure with us the pain and suffering of a progressive, inexorable decline in my health. Secondly, even though I had and still have the greatest regard for my colleagues and know that the respect, affection, and admiration are mutual, I realized intuitively that their knowledge of my illness could destroy my professional life at the medical center.

Let me share some of the reactions of my professional colleagues, beginning with an account of the behavior of my personal physician. To confirm the diagnosis, I traveled to a prestigious medical center renowned for its experience with ALS. The diagnostic and technical skills of the people there were superb, and more than matched the reputation of the institution. The neurologist was rigorous in his examination and deft in reaching an unequivocal diagnosis. My disappointment stemmed from his impersonal manner. He exhibited no interest in me as a person, and did not make even a perfunctory inquiry about my work. He gave me no guidelines about what I should do, either concretely—in terms of daily activities—or, what was more important, psychologically, to muster the emotional strength to cope with a progressive degenerative disease. Stetten recently described his experience after receiving a diagnosis of progressive macular degeneration: "No ophthalmologist has mentioned any of the many ways in which I could stem the deterioration in the quality of my life."[1] The only thing my doctor did offer me was a pamphlet setting out in grim detail the future that I already knew about too well. He asked to see me in three months, and I was too polite or too cowed to ask him why—what benefit was there for me to make the journey again? I still recall that the only time he seemed to come alive during our interview was when he drew the mortality curve among his collected patients for me. "Very interesting," he said. "There's a break in the slope after three years." When, a few months later, I read an article by him in which he emphasized the importance of a compassionate and supportive role for the physician caring for the patient with ALS, I wondered whether he had been withdrawn because I was a physician.

By the fall of 1979 I was walking with a limp; I countered the queries I received in every corridor by saying that I had "a disk." This was not threatening to my colleagues, who proffered advice on how to deal with it and regaled me with their own back problems. I was still a full member of the fraternity, in excellent standing. By early 1980, however, the limp was worse, and I now held a cane in my right hand. The inquiries ceased and were replaced by a very obvious desire to avoid me. When I arrived at work in the morning I could see, from the corner of my eye, colleagues changing their pace or stopping in their tracks to spare themselves the embarrassment of bumping into me. This dramatic change in their behavior occurred when it became common knowledge that David Rabin had ALS. I state with total conviction that my colleagues never meant to hurt me. On the contrary, I was *of* Vanderbilt, and they grieved for me, yet were unable to express their grief.

As the cane became inadequate and was replaced by a walker, so my isolation from my colleagues intensified. I recognize that my own behavior and personality may have contributed to the situation: I am gregarious and, I believe, warm with people; I also value my independence. I did not call a press conference to announce that I had ALS; I did not raise a banner asking for help; rather, I continued to do my work insofar as I was able. Did that put them off? Did they reason, "He wants to pretend that everything is normal, so let's play his game"? How often, as I struggled to open a door, would I see a colleague pretending to look the other way? On the other hand, why was it so natural for the non-physicians—the technicians, the secretaries, the cleaning women—to rush to open the door for me, even if it was the door to the men's toilet? I can only guess that my colleagues thought it would embarrass me if they offered help. How wrong they were, and how distorted their reasoning—accepting help is preferable to sustaining a fracture.

One day, while crossing the little courtyard outside the emergency room, I fell. A longtime colleague was walking by. He turned, and our eyes met as I lay sprawled on the ground. He quickly averted his eyes, pretended not to see me, and continued walking. He never even broke his stride. I suppose he ignored the obvious need for help out of embarrassment and discomfort, for I know him to be a compassionate and caring physician. In trying to understand the behavior of my colleagues I recall an experience I had when I was at Hopkins. I had worked with a splendid physician, Dr. Mason Lord. While still young he developed a brain tumor and he lingered for six or seven months. I always thought up a dozen good reasons to avoid visiting him. Finally, I convinced myself that he really wanted to see only his close friends and family. Of course, I was merely rationalizing. We knew and liked each other, and I failed to go to see him because I would be uncomfortable—not he. I remember my sense of futility when I attended his funeral, because by then it was too late to comfort Mason Lord.

There are so many ways colleagues can help a sick physician. I have learned that the Vanderbilt community admired my ability to continue, in spite of my illness, to function, to maintain my lecture schedule, to write grants and have them awarded, to write papers and have them accepted. The school established an annual lectureship in my name, and my family and I were very moved by this expression of respect and acknowledgment. In the light of this, I may seem ungrateful, and my sense of isolation may seem unwarranted. Nonetheless, continuing personal contact with my colleagues has been rare. I have been working at home for the past year—an arrangement made possible through the consistent and unflagging support of my department chairman. A group of physicians, nurses, and technicians come on a regular basis to work with me. But very few of the physicians with whom I am not collaborating have either called, written, or come to visit.

Some of my close relationships with fellow physicians have also deteriorated since my illness. For a friend to maintain interest and empathy for a week or a month was relatively easy; to show sustained concern over three years required a commitment of quite a different order. I have received relatively few telephone calls or letters from the scores of colleagues I have met in more than twenty years of academic life: former fellows and students, fellow members of study sections, faculty members at numerous medical schools where I have lectured. I hear indirectly about their concern; however, the definitive step of writing me a letter of support is more than the majority can manage. Why this deafening silence? Perhaps it is because we, as physicians, are the healers. We dispense treatment, counsel, and support; and we represent strength. The dichotomy of being both doctor and patient threatens the integrity of the club. To this fraternity of healers, becoming ill is tantamount to treachery. Furthermore, the sick physician makes us uncomfortable. He reminds us of our own vulnerability and mortality, and this is frightening for those of us who deal with disease every day while arming ourselves with an imagined cloak of immunity against personal illness.

We can all recall times when we stood by while a fellow physician behaved irrationally or became frankly psychotic. Most of us are aware of colleagues who are abusing alcohol or drugs. Usually, we delicately ignore the obvious until disaster overtakes the unfortunate physician. I was glad to read in a recent issue of the *Journal* that Vanderbilt is taking steps to help alcoholic physicians.[2] I remember a sensitive and capable psychiatrist at Hopkins who was subject to manic-depressive episodes. His colleagues and I observed the development of manic behavior. We did not intervene, and shortly thereafter his body was found hanging from the ceiling in his hospital office.

It would be erroneous and unfair to say that all physicians avoid and neglect their sick colleagues. In my own case, there are several who have been doggedly and unflinchingly helpful to my family and me. "You have the illness," one friend told me, "but we are in this together." He meant it, and he has followed through with action consistently, to this very day. Although he has a family, a thriving practice, and many interests, he never hides behind the screen of a busy schedule. It has been the thoughtfulness, concern, and spontaneity of many people like him that has enabled my family and me to face the trials and sorrows of this disease. In fact, some physicians with whom we had very little contact before the illness have come forward in our time of need. There are close friends who live many miles away, yet make the time and incur the expense of coming to visit us frequently. One of my former fellows actually moved into my home and helped me in all kinds of ways, including getting me to and from work for eight months.

This account is not intended as a litany of complaint but as a call to physicians to express the compassion they feel toward sick colleagues. It is also meant to draw attention to our frequent inability as physicians to deal with members of our profession who no longer fit the mold of the compleat healer. Toward these ends, I would like to make some concrete suggestions. First of all, do not ignore your colleague. Greet him. Inquire about his health. Offer him support if he is physically handicapped. Don't assume that he prefers seclusion. Ask to visit him. Don't hide behind the false morality of "respecting his privacy"; if it is inconvenient he will tell you.

Secondly, be conscious of the family and extend your support to them. Make a point of asking how your colleague's spouse is feeling and how he or she is coping. The spouse and the children are suffering at least as much as the victim and need support, encouragement, and acknowledgment of their travail. Do not expose the wife to the "premature-widow syndrome," as some physicians do who encounter my wife and never mention my name or inquire about me at all.

Thirdly, bear in mind that the absence of a magic potion against the disease does not render the physician impotent. There are many avenues that can be helpful for the victim and his family. I am often surprised and moved by the acts of kindness and affection that people perform. Fundamentally, what the family needs is the sense that people care. No one else can assume the burden, but knowing that you are not forgotten does ease the pain.

References

1. Stetten, D.J. Coping with blindness. *N. Engl. J. Med.* 1981; 305:458-60.

2. Spickard, A., Billings, F.T., Jr. Alcoholism in a medical-school faculty. *N. Engl. J. Med.* 1981; 305:1646-8.

THE PARIAH SYNDROME: THE SOCIAL DISEASE OF CHRONIC ILLNESS

David Rabin and Pauline L. Rabin

Pariah, a member of any low Hindu caste or of no caste; a social outcast.

(The Oxford Universal Dictionary, Third Edition)

In June 1979, I developed the first symptoms of amyotrophic lateral sclerosis. The public knows this as Lou Gehrig's disease and is aware that it produces a progressive, creeping paralysis of all the muscles of the body. From the time that the diagnosis was confirmed, my wife and I, who are both physicians, were aware of the implications and the catastrophic course which the disease was likely to take. Today, three years later, these dreaded effects have become a reality. However, what we did not fully appreciate was that ALS, or for that matter any chronic incurable illness, also induces a social disease. Patients and their families become pariahs, cast off by many in society who are unable to face them. Thus, they contend not only with their illness but also with the response it evokes.

I would like to share a few personal anecdotes to illustrate our experience. I had been invited to participate in a conference in San Marino scheduled for October 1980. The invitations were extended to about fifty scientists, physicians, and biologists, most of whom I had known for years. Many of these people had been guests at our medical shcool and in our own home. By the time the conference was to be held, I was walking with a severe limp and needed a cane to stabilize my balance. It was by then common knowledge in medical circles that I had ALS. I vacillated about participating in the meeting but finally said to my wife, "This is likely to be the last conference that I will be able to attend. Most of the speakers are good friends, and I think I'd enjoy being with these people one more time." So we decided to go. The experience was little short of a catastrophe for me and my wife. San Marino is not much bigger than its famous postage stamps. The speakers were all housed in the same hotel, had their meals in the same dining room, travelled on the same bus to the conference hall, and spent their leisure time in the same small lounge. This was togetherness. Yet, despite the physical proximity, my wife and I might have been on a desert island. People walked past us with eyes averted or were suddenly mesmerized by the floor. The dining room had a long, narrow, rectangular shape, and for reasons of convenience we were seated early and of course chose the table nearest the door. As the other guests came in to dinner, they literally made a beeline to the corner of the room most distant from ours. If eye contact was unavoidable, there would be a hurried "Hello, David" and off the person would go, almost jet propelled.

Now, I should make one thing clear. In October 1980, my legs were weak, but I had full use of my arms and my speech was unimpaired. While I was seated, it was not possible to identify me as a sick person. What frightened people away was, I suppose, the knowledge that I had an incurable illness. To be charitable, we could say that this was threatening to them and caused them discomfort. To be candid, it was nothing short of brutal treatment. Indeed, had it not been for a few friends at the conference who made a point of sitting with us, of helping me up, and of showing some basic human concern, I don't think my wife and I would have been able to keep our sanity. I still look back on those three days as hell. Somehow we found the strength to drive back to Rome, board a plane, and return home.

About a year after this, the twenty-fifth reunion of our medical school class was to be held. Since so many of our class were living in the USA, it was decided to hold a reunion in New York City. When we were initially approached fifteen months earlier, my wife and I were enthusiastic, but we told the organizer that our attendance would be dependent on my state of health at that time. By October 1981, I had lost the use of all four limbs and was having some trouble with speech and swallowing. Any travel was totally out of the question. Our absence was conspicuous. To our disappointment, only one member of our class who attended the New York reunion called to inquire about my health and expressed his concern and care.

We do not wish to leave the erroneous impression that everyone has behaved towards us in this way. On the contrary, we have been extremely fortunate in having a solid and consistent support system including immediate family, close friends, and some colleagues. It is nevertheless true to say that many people, physicians and non-physicians whom we saw quite regularly before my illness, broke off all social contact with us. We went to some lengths to preserve our broad circle of friends by inviting them to musical evenings in our home. We never heard from many of those people again.

The message was quite clear—my illness had resulted in the irrevocable cancellation of what Susan Sontag has called "the passport of the healthy." Lacking this, my family and I were excluded by a rather large group of people. We had been reclassified as pariahs, social outcasts. This imposed an additional burden on us. Although our professional experience taught us that the phenomenon was surely generic, it nevertheless inexorably damaged our self-esteem. We could not escape the feeling that we must in some way be responsible. But there was another aspect for which it was hard to blame ourselves. This was the failure of acquaintances and friends to even inquire about me when they met my wife or children. A striking example of this occurred after my daughter and I had collaborated on an article on boxing. The class presented their projects at an open house for parents. People who had known me for years and knew I was sick engaged my daughter in conversation about the article but never asked her about her father. My wife has had numerous similar encounters. We have called this the premature-widow syndrome since the patient seems to have become a nonperson.

After months of reflection, we decided that if we were outcasts we were so involuntarily. We also reasoned that if we felt this way so, too, have others. In August 1982, we published an article in the *New England Journal of Medicine* describing our social isolation from fellow physicians. The response was electric.

Hundreds of letters poured in from all over the world—from physicians and lay people, from sick people and their families. The letters were heartbreakingly alike. Over and over again people wrote, "This is precisely what happened to us. We thought we were to blame in some unknown way. What a relief to know that we were not treated in a uniquely cruel manner." A physician who had cancer and was receiving chemotherapy summarized his experience by this statement, "When I walked into the hospital the attitude and demeanor of my colleagues screamed out to me that sick physicians should use the 'tradesmen's entrance.' "

With the author's permission, I would like to share an especially poignant letter. "I am a thirty-three-year-old physician and have experienced many of the things you described in your article. As a result of a rare congenital disease (Marfan's syndrome), I have had to undergo emergency surgery on several occasions during the last two years. Until the first medical crisis I had felt accepted and cared for at the hospital where I worked. Yet when I returned after my initial surgery I experienced what you described so well—the averted eyes, the avoidance by colleagues, the overall lack of expressed sympathy for me and my husband. I, too, realize that these people grieved for me, but I longed terribly for a word of condolence and a direct glance. Shortly thereafter, my husband and I moved, and I tried to start fresh in a residency in Pathology. After only six weeks at work, I again hemorrhaged internally and required abdominal surgery. Although I was admitted to and was operated on at the same hospital as my residency program, no one from the Pathology department called or visited me. Most surprising was the fact that after so much experience I could still be hurt so deeply by the apparent lack of concern of my colleagues. Rereading your article today has eased the pain some, by reminding me that their avoidance is not of *me*, but of their own feelings about illness and death. Thank you for reaching out from your suffering to help me."

A very distressed woman called my wife long-distance immediately after reading the article. Her husband had been in academic medicine in a prominent position at his medical school when he developed ALS. Initially he continued to go in to work. His colleagues avoided him and seemed to deeply resent his presence. She described quite vividly the painful social isolation they experienced for the two years preceding his death. She related that whenever she went to the supermarket former friends would quite overtly try to avoid her. If this ploy failed, they would gush, "My dear, I think of you all the time." She wanted to say, "That's of no help to me"; instead, she would feign politeness to cover up her anger.

Of course, such behavior is not limited to physicians. Every sphere of society in our culture is uncomfortable with chronic illness that defies treatment. One woman told us the following story. The family were members of the Reform congregation and had gotten to know the rabbi quite well while their son was participating in confirmation classes and other proceedings. When her husband became ill, they rather expected that the rabbi would prove to be supportive. He made only one spontaneous visit to their home in the course of a full year. He neither made any offer of support to the boy whose teacher he had been, nor did he encourage any of his congregation to reach out to the famly in distress. The family decided that continued membership was counterproductive. The rabbi, totally oblivious to his dereliction, interpreted their resignation as a sign of financial distress and magnanimously offered to reduce their membership fee!

What accounts for this behavior? Sociologists tell of the overriding desire Americans have for privacy—the American dream is to own a home which is an impregnable castle. The automobile provides personal transport to and from the sanctity of the home. How often have we read accounts of hundreds of commuters each driving their own motor car, windows turned up, a barrier against any intrusion? Our social framework is quite rigidly structured—spontaneous visiting is obsolete. The beautifully kept front lawns of suburbia are remarkable for their absence of people. We sit on our decks or our patios protected by the house as a bulwark against prying eyes. The days of walking to school with friends who live on the same block are long gone. Our children are bused or taken by car to schools remote from their neighborhoods. This premium on privacy seems to have followed a qualitative change in the basic family unit triggered by the industrial revolution. Urbanization and the entry of women into the work force were major factors in shifting the responsibility of caring for the sick from the home. Hospitals became the centers for curing, and failing that nursing homes took on the job of caring. Modern medical insurance has expedited this change by providing reimbursement for expensive institutionalization while covering very limited home nursing care. The net result has been the segregation of the sick from the well. Our lives have become neatly packaged, and we do not have to accommodate to the illness and infirmity of others in our daily schedule. The blind, the deaf, and the handicapped are housed in special enclaves which obviate any need to know how to relate to these people. We take pains to segregate even those who are at risk for developing illness. Thus, we have created retirement centers which offer advantages to the elderly but also serve to isolate them.

Our vision of the spectrum of life experience has narrowed. This has been fortified by the emphasis the mass media place on youth and vitality. Our recent preoccupation with the body beautiful has inadvertently restricted the range of what is deemed acceptable.

Many writers have pointed out that the present generation of Americans is spared exposure to the process of dying. Most deaths occur in hospitals—professionals who are strangers attend the dying person. Funeral services are conducted in the sterile atmosphere of a chapel with soft organ music in the background. We are spared the reality and finality of the open grave. Phillippe Aries has pointed out that, whereas death was once accepted as part of the natural life cycle, attitudes have markedly changed in the twentieth century. Lies began to surround the process of dying, which was seen as something shameful and forbidding. The motivation for this deception was originally a desire to spare the sick person. This was transformed into "an interdict of death," a means of sparing society the anxiety which thoughts of death arouse. In fact, Geoffrey Gorer and others have observed that death has replaced sex as the forbidden topic of our times. Kübler-Ross and her disciples have attempted to reverse this trend. In their writings they have defined five emotional stages experienced by the dying person. Paradoxically, this may have served to increase the isolation of the sick person; a prevalent notion seems to be that dying people working through the Kübler-Ross syllabus are very special and their privacy should be respected.

It is therefore not at all surprising that persons from our culture are totally unprepared when they encounter

illness in what for them seems an inappropriate setting, such as at work, at the supermarket, or at a scientific meeting. Sick people should be in the confines of a
hospital. We know the protocol of acceptable behavior
in this environment. The clergy are comfortable visiting the sick in the hospital and physicians are comfortable making ward rounds. However, outside the legitimate boundaries of a medical center encounters with
sick people are fraught with uncertainty and ambiguity. And because the issues seem so threatening and
discomforting most people simply avoid them. "What
can I possibly say?" they ask. Feelings of frustration,
guilt, and yes, even anger, crystallize towards the sick
person who in the words of anthropologist Robert
Murphy is becoming progressively worse and has the
bad taste to do it slowly.

These current attitudes, so deeply ingrained, will be
hard to alter. One hopeful trend is the increasing willingness of patients with cancer and other chronic
illness to tell their stories, such as Jory Graham's *In the
Company of Others* and Martha Lear's *Heart Sounds*.
Also, the medical profession is reexamining its approach
to patients with chronic disease, and this may spawn
sensitive education programs on illness that will not be
overly sentimental or exploit tragedy. Fundamentally,
however, the problem will not be resolved until the sick
and the well are once more sharing the same space, and
disability will no longer be so strange and may therefore be easier to accept. The question is how will this
happen? Perhaps with the recognition that institutional care is neither good for society nor for the
patient. Society pays a tremendous price fiscally, socio-
logically, and psychologically, and the sick are separ-
ated from their families at the very time when they
most need their support.

The number of residents in nursing homes in the United States has rapidly increased over recent years, reaching 1.3 million in 1978, and is projected to approach 2 million by the year 2000. Nursing home costs were $21 billion in 1980 and if current trends continue will reach $90 billion by 1990. This is a staggering sum which exceeds the entire budget of many countries, and indeed there is no warranty that our economy can sustain these expenditures. Is our society immutably locked into this program or can we devise alternatives to institutionalization of the majority of these people? Those families who wish to care for a chronically sick relative face formidable difficulties when both husband and wife are working. It is therefore necessary to seek some compromise. The program fostered by the hospice movement provides a viable alternative. This philosophy, with its emphasis on home, family, and self-help, provides a means of reintegrating into the fabric of society the phenomenon of dying. The hospice can help the family by arranging for adequate nursing care and household help. They can also provide a support system by way of trained volunteers who will regularly visit those who are homebound or alone for long periods of time.

Can our modern society meet the challenge of dealing compassionately with chronically ill persons? We have struggled with other forms of discrimination and are learning to overcome racism, sexism, and age-ism. Awareness of our prejudice and fear could form the basis of a humanistic approach to the disabled and chronically sick.

CREDO FOR CREEPING PARALYSIS: COGITO ERGO SUM

Pauline L. Rabin and Roni C. Rabin

Three years ago my husband developed the initial symptoms of amyotrophic lateral sclerosis (ALS). The diagnosis was determined clinically and unequivocally confirmed by electromyography. We were devastated by the diagnosis. The full implications were immediately realized since we are both physicians. The course that the illness followed was straight out of a textbook. Stiffness of the legs was followed by weakness. Footdrop developed first on the left, then on the right, and thereafter the disease process progressed inexorably to paralysis of the lower limbs. Weakness of the hands led quickly to global wasting of the small muscles and loss of function of the upper limbs. The paralysis extended more proximally resulting in total quadraplegia. Bulbar symptoms followed with wasting of the tongue, dysarthria, dysphonia, and dysphagia.

The most consistent response I have had from physicians who would discuss the illness with me left me shocked and confused. A neurologist discussing the diagnosis with me said, "It's too bad that this terrible illness spares the brain. David will know exactly what is happening to him to the very end." Another comment was, "What a pity that ALS is not like Alzheimer's." This conveyed to me an undeniable message: all was hopeless; even the unique sparing of the mind in this disease process would only exacerbate the suffering and torture. My purpose in writing this article is to refute this prevalent notion and to state, on the contrary, that amid all the suffering of ALS there is but one pillar which supports the patient and his family, and that is the preservation of intellectual function.

I will describe my experience over the past three years in the hope that this may help physicians to relate to those with ALS in a manner which could optimize the quality of the patient's life. This may prevent the anger and bitterness described by a patient with ALS who condemns the medical profession for its lack of support.[1] It may also prevent the isolation from fellow physicians which my husband and I experienced.[2]

My husband David pursued a very active and successful academic career, his specialty being endocrinology. He was forty-five when the diagnosis was made. Determined to continue to live and work as normally as was possible, David adapted to the physical limitations imposed by the illness. When he could no longer examine patients, he served as a consultant. When he could no longer get to the hospital, he had the laboratory teams come to our home for regular conferences and in this way he was able to direct an active research program. In an era when support for research was difficult, David completed three proposals, all of which were funded. When he could no longer write, he dictated manuscripts, grant proposals, and reviews for the journals on whose editorial board he continued to serve. As his voice weakened, he learned to respond as briefly and succinctly as possible in any scientific dialogue. The fruits of his work in the past three years are testimony to the capacity of man to function despite severe and progressive physical deterioration as long as he retains what is unique to *Homo sapiens*, namely his intellect. Thus, during the past three years, David's group has pioneered work in male contraception and has made important contributions to the understanding of glucose and amino acid metabolism. This month (August 1982) his comprehensive textbook of endocrinology and metabolism, written with T.J. McKenna, M.D., was published. None of this would have been possible without the support, encouragement, and sensitivity of his close colleagues.

My husband's story is not unique. He had a wonderful role model in his own field, Fuller Albright. Albright suffered from severe paralysis agitans and eventually was unable to walk and spoke with the greatest difficulty. His colleagues listened patiently to decipher his almost unintelligible speech. Albright confided to a close friend that he could withstand all his physical disabilities. What depressed him, however, was when people became impatient with his speech, thereby denying him the dignity of an intellectual contribution. The tragedy of Fuller Albright was that unsuccessful surgery deprived him of his wonderful brain.[3]

There are few more dramatic testimonials to the indomitable power of the mind than the story of Franz Rosenzweig, the famous German Jewish theologian. At age thirty-five progressive paralysis set in, and he soon lost his mobility and power of speech. Confined to his home for seven years before his death, he continued intellectual and literary activities. Rosenzweig's concepts have had a profound influence on philosophical and theological thought.[4] Another example is that of the British physicist Stephen Hawking, who has been a victim of ALS for many years.[5] He has actively continued with his mathematical analysis of space and time which have earned acclaim as the work of a rare and authentic genius. I suspect that Rosenzweig and Hawking and many others similarly afflicted have had fulfillment in being able to function intellectually despite progressive, creeping paralysis. I know that David experiences a great sense of satisfaction and contentment in his meaningful academic contributions.

David is keenly aware of the progression of his illness and he grieves over the multiple and continuing losses in function that he sustains. These are the inevitable consequences of being fully alert and conscious. We do not deny them—we mourn them together, but there is compensation in the ability to participate in social and family life. Friends visit often, and we have very heated debates on current international and local events. We have been able to host chamber music concerts on a regular basis, giving David the opportunity to hear fine performances in the company of friends who share a love of music. The suffering of the last three years has also markedly been counterbalanced by the joy given us by our four children. We take as evidence of normal family life arguments and contrary opinions espoused by our children.

People ask me how I have managed to deal with the situation. I have managed because of David and with his help and the constant support of our children, family, and friends. David's pre-illness optimistic personality pervades our home. His open mind and willingness to discuss any subject however painful has enabled us to carry on with our lives. Together we rejoice in his success and achievements just as we share his pain and anguish. As a family we would not have been consoled by a paralyzed and demented David. Certainly, we would not have fared better; neither would he.

I urge my fellow physicians not to abandon patients who are physically disabled. In my opinion, the most important therapy for ALS is the encouragement the physician can give his patient. The physician should prepare the patient for the ordeals that lie ahead and help him to cope with each physical loss as it becomes manifest. Together with his doctor, the patient can devise ways to use the brain long after the muscular paralysis sets in. As one example, when David lost the function of his hands, he was no longer able to read independently. An automatic page turner revolutionized his life and enables him to read prodigiously. Victims of ALS can take heart in the motto *cogito ergo sum*, which I freely translate, "I can think, therefore I am able to function."

References

1. Carus, R. Motor neurone disease: a demeaning illness. *Br. Med. J.* 1980; 280:455-456.

2. Rabin, D., Rabin, P.L., Rabin, R.C. Compounding the ordeal of ALS. Isolation from my fellow physicians. *N. Engl. J. Med.* 1982; 307:506-509.

3. Howard, J.E. Fuller Albright: the endocrinologists' clinical endocrinologist. *Perspect. Biol. Med.* 1981; 24:374-381.

4. *Encyclopedia Judaica*, Vol. 14. Jerusalem, Israel: Keter Publishing House, 1978; 299-303.

5. Ridpath, I. Awesome theories in a wheelchair. *Science Digest* 1978; 84:46-48.

CHEMOTHERAPY FROM AN INSIDER'S PERSPECTIVE

Kenneth H. Cohn

This paper is based on my experience of receiving chemotherapy from November 1980 to July 1981. I was well until October 15, 1980, when I discovered a 3 cm mass in my left mid-neck. Apart from intermittent pruritus and an intertriginous fungus infection at the end of August 1980, I had had no symptoms. I had not noticed any masses before October 15, and I had not lost weight or experienced night sweats. A sonogram showed the mass to be cystic. With the preoperative diagnosis of cystic hygroma, I underwent a cervical exploration on October 10, 1980, and was informed in the recovery room that the frozen section was malignant. Because of a normal bone-marrow aspiration, as well as a negative computerised tomographic scan of the abdomen and pelvis, I was designated stage IA,

54

diffuse undifferentiated lymphoma. After sperm-banking had been completed I began, on November 17, 1980, a thirty-seven-week course of chemotherapy (including bleomycin, adriamycin, cyclophosphamide, oncovin, dexamethasone, methotrexate, and citro-vorum).

PROBLEMS CONFRONTING PHYSICIANS WHO BECOME PATIENTS

The abrupt change from being a surgical resident to becoming a patient gave rise to six problems:

1. Reaction of Health-care Workers to Their Own Mortality

The first difficulty stemmed from the realization by the health-care team that people of their own age and profession can suffer major illness, which was difficult for them to accept.

2. Inadequate Explanations

Another problem was the physicians' difficulties in dealing with a patient who is also a doctor. They seemed apprehensive about talking down to a patient with medical knowledge. This fear led to incomplete explanations of procedures about to be performed and to the failure to explain what complications to expect. An introductory phrase such as "As you know..." would have smoothed this difficult transition. Physicians who had experienced the difference between doing a procedure and having it done on themselves tended to provide more thorough explanations.

It was upsetting after a lumbar puncture to lie flat in bed for twenty-four hours, take a few ginger steps, and then suffer a pounding headache four days after the initial procedure. After hearing about the complication, the resident who carried out the lumbar puncture said, "That is not surprising; one can suffer spinal headaches any time up to ten days after a lumbar puncture." If I had known that, I would have modified my expectations.

Although I feel that for patients to be compliant with treatment they must be informed about their disease, the physicians seemed to find difficulty in talking to me as a patient rather than as a medical colleague. At the end of August 1981, nearly four weeks after the last dose of chemotherapy, I became dyspnoeic with a PO_2 of 41 mm Hg. That experience did not frighten me because I had previously experienced transient failure of other systems during chemotherapy. At the time of this episode of dyspnoea only my heart, kidneys, and hearing had not been compromised at some time. Yet, as breathing became easier, I became increasingly anxious listening to the residents discuss the contingencies of my case as though they were chatting with a fellow physician in the cafeteria rather than with a patient at the bedside.

There was no more powerful incentive for me to improve my breathing than the threat of an open-lung biopsy.

3. Stereotypes

Fear of being stereotyped made me strive to be a model patient and not complain, for I dreaded hearing that "doctors make the worst patients."

4. Morbid Curiosity

I was aware that I attracted morbid curiosity. Everyone seemed to know that I was a doctor by the time I had come in for my second treatment, even though I had never stepped inside this facility previously.

5. Specialty Differences in Outlook

The fifth problem centered on how different medical specialists gather data. Laboratory evaluation seems to take on more meaning in medicine than in surgery. Because I had operated on patients with appendicitis on the basis of their clinical presentation despite normal laboratory findings, I found it difficult to undergo a bone-marrow aspiration and biopsy to look for a "needle in a haystack."

6. Inside Knowledge

The sixth problem was my difficulty in dealing with my helplessness. Most physicians are bright people who have succeeded in every major task they have undertaken. Our medical knowledge and independent spirit diminish our willingness to surrender to our doctors and interfere with the development of trust.

After taking care of patients with a variety of illnesses, I was unable to dismiss the threat of a side-effect as an abstract concept. Many potential complications about which I was informed before consenting to chemotherapy triggered memories of patients who had had the worst imaginable complications of their diseases.

During the difficult moments of chemotherapy I was encouraged to believe that after the treatments had ended I would be free of permanent side-effects, that my hair would grow back, and that I would not have the dry mouth of radiotherapy or the physical deformity of radical surgery. However, I knew of patients in whom successful treatment of disturbance in one organ system was followed by permanent problems in another.

"Rev up the dialysate" was more than just a joke. It was a constant fear during high-dose methotrexate when I was too nauseated to eat or drink.

Medical students learn that oncology is a relatively young discipline and that until more clinical trials have been done many details concerning treatment will remain empirical and unproven. The insecurity of knowing that the optimum duration of therapy is still uncertain stirs up feelings of anger and mistrust when one's own life is on the line.

THE STRESS OF TERMINATION OF THERAPY

I was expected to receive ten courses of chemotherapy—the number of treatments most often useful in this protocol. I was advised that aggressive treatment was the only way to eradicate lymphoma and that no one ever survived a recurrence. However, three days after completing the eighth course of chemotherapy, I became so debilitated that I could not quicken my pace across the street when the traffic light changed. Even walking up half a flight of stairs made me dyspnoeic. After being told that the chemotherapy seemed to be destroying me physically and psychologically and the patients with stage I disease needed less medicine than those with stage III or IV disease, I was told that I would receive no further chemotherapy.

The news that my treatments were finished produced no elation. I felt that, much as I disliked chemotherapy, my lifeline had been taken away from me. I felt that I had "failed the protocol." This "failure" seemed to take the onus off my physicians, since if a recurrence developed it would be my fault for not having undergone all ten courses of chemotherapy. Not until a colleague told me that I had received at least as much medicine as any patient reported in the literature with my stage of disease and the seven-year survival was 100% for those forty-five patients did I begin to feel more secure.

Moreover, the exhaustion which made it impossible for me even to read a newspaper for more than fifteen minutes at a time also prevented me from undertaking any projects. It was difficult to convey to others that people who have prided themselves on their previous accomplishments regard the level of energy as being as much part of the body as the arms, legs, and senses. Exhaustion precluded accomplishment, enhancing feelings of inadequacy and failure. Although I had been assured and knew intellectually that this energy loss would be transient, the lack of improvement for over three weeks made me feel as though the symptoms were permanent.

My psychiatrists believe that termination is the most important part of psychotherapy and spend months preparing patients for it. I recognized a parallel in oncology because, despite the difficulties which I had encountered in the previous nine months, the month after the last treatment was the most stressful of my life. During chemotherapy I was released from the expectations imposed upon me by myself and by close friends. However, once chemotherapy had ended and convalescence had begun, the borders between what I was doing and what I felt that I should be doing became blurred, and I reacted anxiously to the discovery that my career plans, personal relationships, and living arrangements were in a state of flux.

Resentments and anger which I had thought had been dealt with during the course of chemotherapy were expressed in full force afterwards. For the first time since the beginning of my illness, I was asked not to discuss matters pertaining to chemotherapy at the dinner table, was questioned about the prognosis for twenty-five years from now, and was told that once chemotherapy ended I would not be respected until I was working again.

Clearly, in the months after the end of chemotherapy the patient needs the support and caring of his physician as much as, or more than, at any other time of treatment. I hope that reading this paper will trigger mental alarms whenever oncologists think, "He is cured and does not need me any longer."

COPING WITH CHRONIC ILLNESS

The central point regarding chemotherapy from the standpoint of the patient is that these powerful drugs interfered with body functions which most people take for granted, making me feel as though I had surrendered bodily control to a group of external agents. That helpless feeling, rather than an individual side-effect, was what occasioned the need for the greatest adjustment.

The burden of having to deal with the problems of chemotherapy almost all the time depressed my emotional threshold. Frustrations stemming from situations beyond my control triggered outbursts of rage. Annoyances related to therapy included waiting for the results of blood tests in order to receive chemotherapy and the disappointment of not being able to convey to experts in oncology the expertise which had been acquired from being a chronic patient. Whether the failure of communication concerned side-effects which had not been mentioned previously or the intensity of side-effects about which I had been told already, frustration still resulted. These feelings relate not only to medicine, however, but to the communication of any new experience.

Chemotherapy did not become easier with each successive treatment, merely different. Because of the cumulative toxicity of many drugs, symptoms such as nausea and vomiting became worse rather than better. Receiving therapy every two weeks posed a new set of challenges as soon as I had begun to adjust to the obstacles of the preceding treatment.

My doctors agreed that every chemotherapy cycle was to some extent different. What they failed to realize, however, was that this variability did not allow me to predict the duration and severity of side-effects and led, therefore, to enhanced feelings of helplessness.

Constant uncertainties about my daily health and about my ability to function during therapy made it difficult for me to plan social activities or to make commitments about work schedules. All long-term plans had to amend frequently. Colds which produced fever of up to 101.5°F, severe vomiting and diarrhea which resulted from "common enteric viruses," and superficial fungal infections which persisted as long as four months despite treatment made me feel like a group of candlepins that could be easily knocked down.

It is important to describe the coping mechanisms which for me fostered emotional survival as the chemotherapy promoted physiological survival. Despite the resentment of chronic illness which I directed frequently at my health-care team, I found it comforting to be treated by competent, dedicated professionals. Their skill allowed me to eschew the medical literature on lymphoma and to focus on being a patient. Two items learned from surgical residency also helped me— namely, that the easiest way to deal with unpleasant situations is one day at a time and that one can function at less than 100% efficiency.

Cancer has been called a social disease because inevitably it involves other people as well as the patient. Being in a stable, loving relationship and having several close friends and family members with whom I could share my experience helped immeasurably. So I did my work, both because it was stimulating and because it allowed me to feel productive.

Exercise allowed me to maintain my physical condition and to rebound quickly from the side-effects of chemotherapy most of the time. I nicknamed swimming "hydrotherapy" because it renewed my feelings of control over my body, promoted self-esteem, and helped dissipate tension and anger.

Crises improve one's ability to deal with helplessness, sharpen one's focus on important life issues, and result in a sense of accomplishment, once resolved. The opportunity for personal growth during chemotherapy can and should be conveyed to patients, because the heightened self-esteem which results from that growth will increase patients' stamina during treatment and diminish the likelihood of their discontinuing therapy prematurely.

The reasons why I regard the time spent in chemotherapy as disruptive but not unproductive stem not only from having received treatment for a previously fatal disease but also from the knowledge which I have gained about the art of patient care as a result of having been ill. In many ways, my experiences have changed the care which I now offer to patients. As my veins become increasingly scarce, mobile, and collapsible, I sometimes had to be needled as many as five times because laboratory technicians would not listen when I said that "Vacutainers" did not work any more;

and so I now understand patients' anger when they feel that their warnings are not being heeded. Also, I now try to avoid strongly worded explanations to patients for fear of committing myself to a position which I would later regret.

THE LESSONS OF CHEMOTHERAPY

I learned six major lessons during chemotherapy:

1. Surprise spits in the eye. Any event that occurs unpredictably, regardless of the cause, should be expected to produce feelings of helplessness and outrage. The most difficult situations for me to deal with were not the diagnosis of lymphoma or the initial hair loss, because they were events for which I was prepared. The most challenging events were a grand-mal seizure, a toxic reaction to phenytoin, the second episode of alopecia, and the stresses of terminating chemotherapy, because they were events that surprised me. The only times I considered terminating chemotherapy prematurely were during these "surprises," because each one made me feel as though the light at the end of the tunnel represented an oncoming train rather than daylight. Intermittent desire to stop chemotherapy reflected my inability to cope with the unpredictable side effects of treatment, not an objective calculation of the amount of medicine necessary for cure. Wigs, physical activity, and patient education are ways of counteracting helplessness which chemotherapy causes.
2. Anger is a very common response to the multiple challenges of being a patient, but when directed outwards (preferably not at those who care for one) it

fosters a renewed sense of energy. The pride which resulted from my accomplishments during chemotherapy helped supply the stamina necessary to endure treatments.

3. The alternating sickness and health made me feel as though I were riding a physiological roller coaster. Nevertheless, a 50% day following a 10% day always felt like a tremendous improvement rather than being measured against my presickness efficiency.

4. Any event which disrupted my equilibrium increased my feelings of helplessness and reduced my ability to tolerate the frustrations of daily existence.

5. The disruption which resulted from my illness produced opportunities for personal growth which I had not considered previously.

6. Because of the unknown effects of chemotherapeutic agents on gametes, therapy in men should be delayed two weeks if possible to permit sperm-banking.

CONCLUSION

I hope this paper will help both patients undergoing chemotherapy and the physicians who care for them. Today's oncologists need to be encouraged to derive feelings of self-esteem and career satisfaction from improving the quality as well as the quantity of their patients' existence. By addressing the emotional problems associated with chemotherapy they can diminish their patients' feelings of abandonment and rage and prevent the despair which patients suffer when made to feel as though they are the only ones having difficulty with therapy. Self-esteem and functional coping mechanisms are undoubtedly prerequisites to accomplishment in people whose physiological health is compromised.

ANGER AS FREEDOM

Jory Graham

Anger is as basic to cancer as fear. It is a normal response to sudden, wrenching, irrevocable change that shatters all our expectations, our plans, and our sense of future.

Even if frustration or bitter disappointment has characterized our lives, most of us will discover that a diagnosis of cancer changes our perspective 180 degrees. Now life is precious, and God, O God, we don't want it taken from us, now or ever.

The unrecognized calamity of cancer is not that we may die of it, but that we are so likely to lose our autonomy to it. From the time our doctor, or a surgeon we've just met, says, "I want you in the hospital on Wednesday," we are expected to behave like patients, quietly acquiescing in the doctor's, the medical team's, and the hospital's rules. Beginning in the hospital admissions office, the message is clear: "The little plastic band [placed] on the arm of the patient as part of the admitting process [is] an expression of property rights.... It means we now take possession of you."[1]

Hospitals exist to heal people, but in order to be treated in a hospital every patient must fit into a pre-existing slot. Strangers take over: doctors, nurses, aides, technicians, orderlies—mainly cool and self-distancing personnel, oblivious to the depersonalizing effect they have on us. In a teaching hospital with a cancer center, teams of specialists, medical students, and a full house staff (interns and residents) take even fuller control of our bodies and our lives. We are expected to be part of the team, but only in a passive, compliant role.

To hospital personnel, our fear, our insecurity, our overwhelming feeling of having received a death-sentence are commonplace. House staff and nurses *expect* cancer patients to be frightened and anxious, but all too often their understanding of fear and anxiety is superficial. They do not, or cannot, allow themselves to feel what we now feel: the nausea and terror having been abruptly torn loose from our moorings to confront the world's most feared disease.

So, except for the impersonal touch of physical examination, or a change of dressings, we are like untouchables to the hospital personnel. In their own eyes, they are correctly professional. They signal they want no involvement. The message, alas, comes when we are most vulnerable, most in need of expressions of love and concern.

We resent the arbitrary obliteration of self, but because we are weak and, perhaps, in postsurgical pain, we are rarely able to voice our feelings. I remember only a few occasions when I could use my anger to effect change. One was during a bone scan, a long procedure in which a patient, semiconfined by sandbags, had to lie motionless under a heavy metal scanner which passed with paleolithic slowness over his body and then back again and yet again.[2] This enormous, disk-like piece of equipment was less than an inch above one's nose and, because it moved slowly, most patients were asked if they suffered from claustrophobia. If the answer was yes, as mine was, the technician monitoring the scan usually sat near enough that the patient could feel his presence, and usually offered reassuring comments during the scan. Conversation between patient and technician was not permitted, because talking created head motion.

On this particular occasion, I was wretchedly nauseated and in considerable pain. Lying flat on my back, motionless, for the necessary twenty-three minutes was close to unbearable. The technician, a young man, disappeared as soon as he knew the scanner was functioning properly; a young woman I assumed was another technician seated herself somewhere out of my sight and proceeded to rattle through a newspaper.

My claustrophobia mounted. My pain was intense. Her lack of concern infuriated me. I yearned to knock the newspaper out of her hands and yell, "Pay attention to me, *pay attention.*" Instead, I had to use most of those twenty-three minutes to convince myself that I was not going to suffocate. The balance of the time I spent wondering how to use the experience to help patients who would come after me.

When the scan ended, I swallowed my anger and asked the young woman how long she'd been working in the department. She was a technician in training; this was her second week. "You know," I said, "you could do more for your patients and also make the job rewarding for yourself."

"I could?"

"Yes, you could. Try that scanner on a dry run with yourself as the patient. Learn how frightening it is to lie under it. Lie there immobile, silent, scared, alone. I felt alone because you buried yourself in your newspaper. I needed some concern from you. That would have been comforting. You are part of the healing process, you know."

A small thing, but I got through to her. Later I even laughed at Jory Graham, crusader for cancer patients, who on this occasion thought she had scored a tiny victory.

This incident occurred during my third year as a cancer patient. By then I had been hospitalized seven or eight times and was no stranger to the department of radiation therapy, or to diagnostic radiology, or to nuclear medicine (where I reported for scans). I was no longer intimidated by the hospital system, and I felt entitled to speak out. Yet from the start I was outraged by it, because it forces patients to initiate overtures of friendship to medical personnel at the time they feel least capable of reaching out.

I wanted that student-technician to understand how much good she could do by reaching out; I wanted everyone in the hospital system to understand and acknowledge by word and gesture the human needs of cancer patients. I saw the unnecessary frustration and despair brought into play each time the system ignored those needs. Patients must have something with which to build hope; optimism ("You must be optimistic," say the doctors) cannot replace feelings of depression and defeat easily, if at all.

The inhospitality of hospitals is felt by many patients. But those with a fractured bone, a hernia, or a painful gall bladder have enormous advantages. For one thing, they know their pain will subside and vanish as their bodies heal. For another, they know they will soon return to the normal routines of their lives. They may rail at the hospital system, but they can tolerate it, because their stay is relatively short and almost without fear.

A hospitalized cancer patient has none of these securities. Hospitalization alone does not ensure healing and in many instances it marks another setback. For a cancer patient, it is often an ordeal beyond the comprehension of his physician, the house staff, his family, and his friends. He cannot talk about it to any of them because, in one way or another, all these people have demonstrated that they do not want to listen to minute details of feelings he can only timidly express. Further, they are trying so hard to reassure him, and so much of the reassurance sounds false, that he feels conned and even more insecure. Are they withholding information about his illness? Are they making decisions for him on the basis of their greater knowledge of his condition? What do they know that he isn't being told? What does his doctor mean when he says, "You must be optimistic"? How can anyone feel optimism in the face of what is clearly another battle lost to cancer? The cancer patient is too weak to protest, yet his perceptions are often as keen as his pain, and just as stabbing.

As hospitalized cancer patients, we understand that we are objects of medical care. Once discharged, we often discover we have become objects in our own world, too, where we are now seen as "the terminally ill," or as another "cancer victim." People who sent flowers and get-well cards to us in the hospital now feel they have exhausted these conventional forms of showing concern. Our homecoming removes the distance between us and they feel uneasy with the new closeness. The comfortable relationships we shared before

give way to timidity and awkwardness. How quickly
we come to know the signals of their instant need to
retreat. And though we feel like pleading, "Stay, stay,
I've come back from the brink and I'm weak and I'm
weary and lonely and I need you," we have pride, and
dignity, and a much greater understanding of their
feelings than they have of ours, and so we are tactful
and let them go.

What is harder to release, because there is no outlet
for it, is our anger at their illogical fears, at their need to
flee. *Dammit, don't you understand where I've been,
what I've come through, what a triumph it is to be
alive? Can't you understand how I hurt and how you
are adding to the hurt? I didn't ask to have cancer, but I
didn't go looking for it; despite what has happened to
me I'm still me. Come back. There's nothing to fear.
You can't catch what I've got. It's not your life that's at
stake. You're not trapped—I am. You're free to continue
your life just as it is. You're so blessedly* free.

Oh, if only we could be free again, free of the hateful
disease and the fear and anger and despair that it
brings, over and over again. We nearly strangle on
emotions; together, they create untold suffering and
demoralization. We so turn to God, the last resort for
many of us who have been remote from God since
childhood. And all of us ask God one question: Why me?

*Why me, and not that bum down the block who beats
his wife and terrifies his kids? Why me, and not that
power-drunk vice-president who heads my department?
Why me, just on the edge of achievement, rather than
the crazed old woman who fishes about in the garbage
cans along the alley for the discards of our meals? Why
me, and not the really evil people in this world?*

*Who sent this gnawing worm into me, You or the
devil? What am I—a sinner? All right, I'm a sinner. I*

*was impatient with my mother when her brain began
to dull. Yes, and angry with her for becoming senile and
incompetent. I despised my weak father. I've belittled
my wife—and cheated on her. But get cancer for these,
the acts of men everywhere?*

We fumble through a Bible. *Here it is, here in St. John
it says, "If ye shall ask anything in my name, I will do
it." Do it. Cure me. I ask You. I beg you. And tell me,
why* me?

In July 1977, I wrote "Coming to Terms with 'Why
Me?' " It was my third column for the *Chicago Daily
News*, the first U.S. newspaper to run my column. I
wrote it during the week I was moving from an apart-
ment I loved. I was in a building that had turned con-
dominium, and in the face of cancer, I could not afford
to buy it. My father refused to lend what I would have
needed to make the down payment. He thought it was
insane to buy real estate when you were doomed. I was
tired and ill at the time because of all the radiation I
had been receiving, and moving was a nightmare. I
tried lifting something and felt as if the vertebrae in my
lumbar spine had collapsed. Pain was instant and
excruciating. I had to go for emergency examinations
and x-rays. I was lucky: no bone had compressed and
fractured. But I was incapable of pain-free motion, and
the only release was to lie on the floor and let its hard-
ness mitigate the awful pain.

Lying on the floor, surrounded by packing cases and
the disorder of moving, I worked with my tape recorder
and drafted "Coming to Terms with 'Why Me?' "

"The question is pitiful, unavoidable, and normal," I
told my readers. I had asked it of myself when I first
learned I had cancer—and needed months to forge an
answer.

An answer; there is no *one* answer. Each of us has to

come to terms with *why me?* in our own way. However, I outlined four possible answers.

The first answer to *why me?* originates in Genesis: God has selected this illness for me because of my sin; I am being punished.

A second answer is a late twentieth-century form of paranoia: society is doing this to me. It's our tense, pressured environment. Everything is polluted. Everything is contaminated.

A third answer to *why me?* is a pseudopsychological notion: I have brought this on myself. I'm a failure as a human being and driven by unconscious needs to seek a way out.

A fourth answer is existentialist. The universe is absurd. The tragedies that befall us are a matter of luck. Luck is random. This just happened to catch me.

These are the major choices, and I personally find all but the last of them categorically untrue. To believe that cancer has been aimed at us by a vengeful God is to further burden ourselves with unnecessary guilt. If we are all sinners, how can some of us be selected to suffer while others go free?

Blaming society is simply an extension of a lifetime of blaming everyone else for one's own problems. A paranoid answer is no answer at all.

The idea that we bring about our own disease strikes me as the wildest theorizing from knowledge of psychosomatic medicine. To state that some of us have cancer-prone personalities is not only a cruel accusation but a stupid one. How do these researchers explain cancer in newborn infants? How developed can a cancer-prone personality be at birth?

Fortunately, for every psychologist who insists upon associating a cell disease like cancer with certain adult personality traits, there is a psychiatrist or psycho-analyst who will say, "I wish the notion were true. If it were, we could cure you."

A friend whose young wife died of cancer told me that she had tortured herself wondering if she were respon-sible for her condition. "She was depressed enough just dealing with the cancer," he said, "without having to feel she had brought it on herself. That simply exacer-bated her problems, and the worst of it was, it was so unproven and untrue."

Which brings us to existentialism. I opt for it because it offers hope and also because I believe that our ordered universe is, in many ways, absurd. The way to find meaning in an absurd situation is take some kind of action. My action was a search for a different per-spective on *why me?*, because the question is so loaded with implications of injustice. Since I could not blame God, or myself, or the polluters of our environment, I was confounded—and angry. I didn't know why I had cancer (I still don't), but the unfairness of losing my freedom and my life to it filled me with rage.

One day, though, I tried finding an answer with that old puzzle that represents three rows of three dots each, as follows:

. . .

. . .

. . .

Without retracing your path, you are to draw four con-necting lines that pass through every dot. The problem is *not* solved by drawing a box, like the one below, because this takes five lines.

The solution depends upon your ability to think *outside the box.*

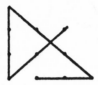

I was tinkering with the solution only because I half recalled it, but my mind was on *why me?* Suddenly it occurred to me to think outside the question, that is, turn the question around and ask, why *not* me? My mind opened instantly.

Why not me? Who am I to be so special that I cannot get cancer? Who am I to be so egocentric as to believe that random luck is for others, but not me? From then on, it was only a matter of time to *it is me*, and, *what am I going to do now?* With this question came a feeling of enlightenment and a sense of power.

We cease feeling trapped and powerless once we recognize that we can still make decisions and have choices. The choices may be radically limited by the extent of our illness, and the decisions may often seem meager, but knowing we have them to make can alleviate some of our sense of powerlessness. This is true for those of us who were heavy smokers and have cancer of the lung or larynx; and for those of us who continued to work in asbestos plants long after we clearly understood the carcinogenic dangers there. We may feel we're being punished, but the truth is that smoking, or remaining in the asbestos plant, was an action we chose freely. The risk was a risk we were willing to take. We gambled. We lost.

Do we now destroy all meaning and any pleasure in the time that is left by wallowing in self-hatred? No, we do not. We need to use our decision-making ability to help our families and friends through the ordeal that lies ahead. That's what we still can do, and that's what matters now.

I made the decision to use the rest of my life on behalf of cancer patients everywhere. Along with many of my readers, I also decided that no hour alone or with those I love would be wasted in self-pity or guilt. I said to my readers, we simply have no time to waste. The time we do have is for reaching out, giving, building our own legacy of courage and concern for others.

If we are not to sink into chronic depression and helpless anger, we have to go beyond the futile attempt to find an answer to *why me?* to acceptance of the fact that we have cancer: *I have it. Now what do I do?* This is the decision that will give meaning and significance to the rest of our lives, despite physical limitations, recurrent frustration, and fear.

In accepting cancer as the probable cause of my death, I realize that I now have nothing but my life to lose. I am free to speak out, to crusade for the rights of cancer patients everywhere. The fact that I have a column means only that I have a wider audience to reach. Yet my voice is nothing if it is not joined by yours.

The image of a cancer patient retreating from the mainstream is often accurate. Sometimes an individual is pressured into retreat by the discrimination he encounters. Often times, he is so ashamed of having cancer, or so terrified of it, that he creates a wall of silence to hide behind.

I do not accept the image of retreat, and I do not let others dictate the confines of my life. One theme that runs through my newspaper column like a *leitmotif* is the belief that we should not give up before we must; that by our actions, by our behavior inside and outside the hospital, we will change the image of the demoralized, pitiful cancer patient. The dialogue between my readers and me in "A Time for Living" shows repeatedly the courage and determination characteristic of most of the cancer patients I know. The column reinforces their inner strength, their rejection of the cruel attitudes of others, and their affirmation that anger in these situations is justified and can be put to work for us.

I once wrote a strong letter to a man who'd been a close friend but who could not deal with my cancer. I told him to get off his duff and get back to me. Though my letter failed to bring him back, it served another purpose: in writing it, I realized I was not so helpless after all.

I have written more than one column on the meanness inherent in the label "cancer victims,"[3] that odious label used daily by all the media and even by the American Cancer Society. Some members of the media and the ACS are beginning to understand the need to change.

Angered over the ostracism he encountered as a cancer patient, Orville Kelly, a small-town Iowa newspaper editor, founded Make Today Count, a support group, in 1974. Kelly's purpose was "to allow cancer patients and their families an opportunity to come together and discuss their emotional problems." It's not surprising that more than 270 Make Today Count groups are currently active in the United States and other countries.

Equally angry because of the ways the human needs and fundamental human rights of cancer patients are being ignored, I joined with approximately thirty-five caring physicians, lawyers, business men and women, and cancer patients and their families. In 1979, we founded a new issue-oriented national organization: One/Fourth, the Alliance For Cancer Patients And Their Families.[4]

Because almost nobody knows how to handle anger, cancer patients are expected to suppress their anger about the way the disease is destroying their lives. This is unrealistic and unhealthy. Suppressing anger is not the answer—it too often leads to chronic depression and shortened life span[5]—yet the function of healthy expressions of anger is not understood at all.

I was furious when my cancer metastasized and nailed me onto the endangered list. I'd fought hard to win the first round, yet seven months later I had to enter the match again and make an even greater effort, though with little hope of winning more than added time. I was so frustrated, so disappointed, so thwarted because the earlier effort seemed to have been in vain that I lashed out at everyone—and all but drove them away.

Fear that they might not return brought me to my senses. After all, they were not to blame for my disease, and it was unfair to ask them to listen to a long-playing diatribe. I began looking for creative ways to handle anger. I asked my readers to contribute their solutions. My favorite answers are these, from two readers who have become good friends of mine:

Patty Grate wrote that she made a rag bag the size of

a Santa Claus pack. When she becomes so angry that she feels she's "going to kill," she hauls the rag bag into the bathroom and closes the door and the cover to the toilet. "And then I sit on the convenience and tear rags into shreds until the utter stupidity of what I am doing gets to me and I can come out laughing again."

Michael Spekter wrote that he was going to have fourteen-by-sixteen enlargements made of his pathology slides. "I'll mount them as dart boards and hurl darts at the dark areas that show tumors."

A doctor finally suggested to me that I learn to shout, "I hate having cancer." I felt silly and self-conscious the first few times I tried, but I learned to say it to empathetic friends. In a funny way it helps, because it's an honest statement. It does not drive away friends, because it does not blame them for our misfortune. It is a legitimate focus for our very real anger, anger that threatens to get out of hand but is diffused by a simple statement of fact.

Healthy anger gives us vitality. It is a glorious sign that we're far from dead. It makes us fight for our jobs—and pride makes us work twice as hard at them. Healthy anger gives us purpose, challenges us to make new decisions, encourages old ideas: to enroll in the courses we've always wanted to take; to embark on the trip we've always wanted to make; to create the journal that is our legacy to our children and our grandchildren...

> "Do not go gentle into that good night,
> Rage, rage against the dying of the light."[6]

References

1. Mauksch, H.O. The organizational context of dying. In: *Death: The Final Stage of Growth*, ed. Elisabeth Kübler-Ross, (Englewood Cliffs, N.J.: Prentice-Hall, 1975), p. 17.

2. Nuclear medicine now has much newer, faster equipment than this, though it may not yet be in general use.

3. Graham, J. When media insensitivity does harm. Appendix A in *In the Company of Others*. New York: Harcourt Brace Jovanovich, 1982, p. 133-135.

4. One/Fourth addresses the social and human aspects of cancer on a broad scale, complementing the American Cancer Society's work on medical advances against the disease.

5. Derogatis, L.R., Abeloff, M., and Melisaratos, N. Psychological coping mechanisms and survival time in metastatic breast cancer. *J.A.M.A.* 242:1504-1508, 1979.

6. Thomas, D. Do not go gentle into that good night. In: *The Collected Poems of Dylan Thomas* (New York: New Directions, 1946), p. 128.

DOCTORS AND CANCER PATIENTS

Nathan Schnaper, Tamar K. Kellner, and Barbara Koeppel

Today's oncologist is a scientist, a fact supported by his dedication to research and computerized technology. In recent years there has been greater emphasis on the study of the total person and yet, perhaps unfortunately, an increase in specialization. As a by-product of this paradox, the concept of the family doctor is blurred and the patient is cared for by a scientist. This, in itself, is not bad, but it is not enough. The physician-oncologist has to approach his patient with a psychological awareness of himself as well as of the patient.[1]

Much debate has surrounded the issue of cure and care, and their relative importance in healing. Many claim that little attention is given to the latter, while far too much is accorded the former. The problems involved for medical personnel in caring for patients are nowhere more pronounced than with the terminally ill, but the focus, nevertheless, remains on curative questions. This is true despite the fact that a diagnosis of an incurable condition triggers a complex set of patient-family-physician reactions which directly affect these individuals, their interrelationships and roles. In such situations, the "quality of care" becomes crucial. And if the medical helpers, particularly the oncologists, recognize these reactions, their roots and manifestations, they can offer dying patients the support, strength, and dignity they need in this most difficult of times.

The state of death is impossible to conceptualize, and the thought of dying terrifies. Since "being dead" cannot even be imagined, a void evolves only to be filled with superstitions, fantasies, and poetic creations. We know there are several classifications of death: medical death, in which heart action ceases and with it cell nourishment; civil death, when a person has been absent, though perhaps alive, and unheard from for a long period of time, and is declared legally dead; and religious death, which anticipates continuation of life either through transmigration of the soul or hereafter in the kingdom of God. But these are descriptive concepts rather than dynamic ones.

So we grant that any real understanding of death is beyond us. Perhaps in some future scientific age, understanding will be achieved. Not so with dying. The very word evokes pain and apprehension, in the doctor as well as in the patient. The patient fears it for himself and his family. The doctor has similar personal concerns, and also must cope with the problem in his work day after day. How does he react to his patient dying? Does he meet the problem or avoid it? What can he do for the patient? Should he tell the patient? If so, how much? What? How? What can he do to help the patient through this period? This is the task to which the following paragraphs are addressed.

The terminally ill can be patients with nonfulminating, cardiovascular, renal, neurologic diseases or carcinoma; but for the purposes of this discussion, the patient dying of cancer will be used as the model.

THE PATIENT

When patients are confronted with the diagnosis of cancer (the physician's dilemma, to tell or not to tell, will be discussed later) or with symptoms, e.g., a woman finds a lump in her breast, anxiety immediately sets in. Just the word "cancer" instantly evokes terrible thoughts of death, mutilation, emaciation, and the like. Individuals also experience a profound sense of futility, that there is no present or future prospect of resolving the problem.

Enormous stress and a host of mechanisms to deal with it accompany such thoughts. Some of these responses are useful, and lead the individual to take prompt and necessary action. Other reactions, such as denial, often lead to delay which can be critical.

What are the signs of stress? Patients describe an emotional paralysis—they feel initially "stunned," or "fragmented." A great number experience guilt or shame, they believe their illness is related to something they did which was bad; e.g., they were too hostile, unkind (to parents or others), selfish, or sinful. In one study by Finesinger et al., 93 per cent of cancer patients admitted to feeling guilty about getting the disease; in another, 66 per cent said, "It's my fault. I've done something wrong." They are ashamed they have such a "frightful illness." Others feel inferior or inadequate.[2,3]

Besides guilt, patients are caught in a maze of fears that relate to death itself. These take various forms, but the most common, of course, is the fear of the unknown. "I am going to die. What's going to happen to me? Am I going to rot? Will worms eat me when I am buried? Is there a 'final judgment'?"

Next, there are the fears of death that center on loss; of the inevitable separation, being cut off from the nurturing people, whether relatives, mates, children, or parents; of what will be missed, like seeing children graduate from school or get married, the birth of grandchildren, etc.; of the loss of body image—with the high incidence of the disease, most have been exposed at one time or another to the progressive deterioration of others and they fear they too will become wasted as they pass through the various stages of the illness; of the loss of control, similar to the fear experienced by patients about to be anesthetized ("In my weakened state, will I be revealing secrets or saying terrible things I don't want people to know?"); of the inevitable regression and dependency—"Will I be helpless, dependent on others, no longer in control of my life?" In total, a loss of identity.[4]

Once in the dying process, patients do, in fact, become increasingly dependent just as they feared. As a defense against their weakening and subsequent helplessness, patients experience *regression*. During this period, they are in great need of their helpers, particularly their doctors and nurses. They are aware, though unconsciously, that they are more and more passive, dependent, and vulnerable and quite naturally (just as any healthy individual would feel in such a dependent situation) resent those upon whom they have come to rely. But a contradiction arises, as patients feel, again unconsciously, that they must not be resentful, since the helpers are being so nice and trying to cure them. Thus, guilt develops and one encounters patients who are withdrawn, demanding, or irritable.

Another defense marshalled by patients against the

reality of dying, though not so prevalent, is to reject help, to succumb to the inevitable, refusing medications, therapy, etc., preferring to die. Very few, however, are suicidal. Far more common is the opposite behavior, where patients will go to any lengths, e.g., visits to countless specialists (ethical and/or quack) all across the country, or submit to toxic medications and painful procedures to stay alive. Even physicians who say that, if confronted with cancer, they would kill themselves, will rarely follow through when it in fact occurs. To commit suicide is to relinquish denial and thereby hope.

The most effective defense is *denial*, either outright or indirect. With the first, patients protect themselves from the truth by simply negating it. A good example of such behavior is of a physician who has spent his life working with the psychological aspects of cancer and in whom, as fate would have it, a carcinoma developed. He felt that patients should be told—gently, of course. The surgeon who operated on him did not concur with this approach, but respecting the physician's opinions on the matter, decided to inform him. From then on, for the time that he lived, the physician never used the word cancer again. Six weeks before he died, he referred to the medication for his "gall bladder infection." The pills, of course, were meperidine.

A less obvious tack, but one just as effective, is the course of intellectualizing about the disease. By doing this, patients obscure its reality and treat it as if it were history and unrelated to them. They speak of it, their symptoms, their daily blood counts and the like, but only as a subject that is somehow apart from them.

Denial is crucial and cannot be taken away from a patient. Whether patients are "told" or "spared," they know, regardless of whether they are professionals or high school drop-outs. And after they know, in most cases, denial, which is a form of hope, begins. The dilemma this poses for the helpers will be discussed later.

THE FAMILY

Families of the cancer patient play an integral part as the patients move through the different phases of the disease. Their initial reactions to the diagnosis of cancer, as well as to the actual process, directly affect the patients and the helpers.

The most common reactions to the diagnosis that are directed toward the helpers are resentment and/or pressure. The former is aimed at the diagnosing physician and is especially intense when the patient is a child. In some way, the diagnosis is the physician's fault. The anger is "to the messenger rather than the message." The other appears usually in the form of requests that patients not be told "the truth," to "spare" them. This is the result of the families' unconscious guilt for having been spared themselves.

There are simultaneous responses, directed to the patients, as grief begins. Families mourn the anticipated death in a manner similar to that displayed whenever there is a loss, whether separation, family crises, financial catastrophes, etc. There are many forms and phases of grief, which include the initial shock, followed by a period of emotional release, covert hostility, utter depression, physical symptoms, panic, guilt, overt hostility, inability to resume normal activities, waning of mourning, and finally some final resolution and readjustment to reality. Grief may be viewed succinctly as *shock, turmoil,* and *resolution.* The intensity of each state varies, but one aspect is fixed; all things start little and grow big except grief, which begins large, grows small, and in time generally disappears. When the grieving is not resolved, the intervention of a psychotherapist is needed.

To deal with their grief, individuals respond differently. Some move too close to patients, overwhelming them in their unconscious attempt to ward off guilt feelings they may have about their relationship. Others will repeatedly try to advise the physician and patient about the patient's treatment. The opposite behavior is also witnessed where families abandon patients, as if they had already died. This, too, represents an unconscious attempt at self-protection, to lessen the hurt when the death actually occurs. But in both cases, the mourning process comes, regardless.

PHYSICIANS

Physicians, too, bring to the cancer patient their own reactions based on their unique backgrounds, experiences, and personalities. Some of their responses are helpful, others are not. Often, because of their particular personalities and defenses, surgeons and internists (though not oncologists) are uncomfortable or even incapable of treating cancer patients. They reject them completely and turn them over to the residents, or, less blatantly, limit visits to 30 seconds.

They reason that their difficulties in dealing with dying patients stem from personal identification; i.e., that the patient reminds them of a parent or close relative, and an intense doctor-patient relationship is too painful, as it summons forth distressing memories.

What is at stake, in fact, is the physician's sense of

omnipotence, a key component in the personalities of those who have chosen professions in which they derive satisfaction from positions of control (ministers and teachers also fall into this category). When this need is sublimated and channeled into healthy outlets, society benefits. When it is not, however, the situation provokes anxiety in the professional. This is especially apparent with cancer patients, for in many of these cases, physicians are unable to cure and therefore feel they have lost their powers. And, just as patients and families ascribe to physicians magical powers of healing, so too do the "healers" themselves, whose expectations are often just as unrealistic.

Thus the diagnosis may spark the physician's hostility toward the patient, either direct or covert, since the inevitable death threatens his omnipotence. The doctor reasons, "No patient has the right to die when I am the doctor." Angered, some simply avoid the dying patient altogether; others, repressing the hostility, retaliate by using the time with the patient to read mail, make phone calls, or the like.[5]

The threat to omnipotence stems from the physician's unconscious fear that he is accountable for the death. Subconsciously, the doctor concludes, "Since I have the power to cure, I must also have the power to kill." The roots for such rationale are laid in childhood when the infant is, indeed, omnipotent. Infants cry or simply grimace and the parents respond immediately. As children develop and pass through the normal state of ambivalence toward people and objects in their environment, feelings of power are easily transformed into feelings of pain. Wishes are equated to deeds, for children believe that merely wishing the parent "away" (dead), as when the child is being punished by the parent, may elicit the actuality. Such imagined power frightens children, because they believe they will be held accountable, i.e., an eye for an eye. However, in time, if development proceeds normally, the sense of power and ambivalence is sublimated into healthy outlets. Much later, however, when some physicians are faced with the inevitability of their patient's death, they are overcome by guilt. Borrowing from the past, they are again somehow responsible and must separate before "the moment of truth."

Closely akin to the physicians' need for omnipotence is their need to be loved. Patients who are anxious, frustrated, and demanding may cause physicians to feel anxious and unloved. Thus they offer the patients long, elaborate explanations, to cull their favor.[6]

Some physicians are uncomfortable with the heightened closeness that ensues as patients become more dependent. For many, occupying such a pivotal role in their patients' lives is unbearable, as it threatens their need to remain distant, clinical observers—a technique some oncologists find necessary. In such cases, physicians refer their patients to consultants, hospitals, or nursing homes in order to avoid close contact.

Interestingly enough, patients generally remain loyal and rarely complain about such behavior. If they venture a criticism, it is usually tempered with pronouncements about the physician's competence, skill, and dedication.

MANAGEMENT OF THE PATIENT WITH CANCER

Care of the cancer patient is not simply a matter of administering the proper therapeutic and pain medications at the appropriate moment, though this is indeed a part of the task.[7] Rather, the patient's physical and emotional well-being is inextricably linked, and the care provided therefore must account for the whole range of patient-family-helper reactions mentioned above.

Patients with cancer are, of course, special; but they are also similar to all other patients in that they deserve the care afforded the rest. As with others, they should be treated with compassion, with reassurance, and with everything we have in our medical, surgical, and radiotherapeutic armamentarium. Because of the nature of their illness and some of the methods of treatment, those with terminal disease may be, and have a right to be, irritable.

This is not to say that the oncologist must be all-accepting and permissive with his patient. One is not suddenly holy or good simply because he is dying. One dies as one has lived. If one has been flexible in dealing with life, he will cope in a cooperative way. In a sense, he can "live with cancer." If one has been rigid, arrogant and mean in the past, he will continue to be so during the process of dying.[8] Physicians, however, need not or must not love or hate such patients; they must treat them. The oncologist does not have the advantage of establishing, prior to the onset of the disease, solid doctor-patient relationships upon which trust through the very difficult period may build. Nonetheless, it becomes crucial that he have insights into the personal interactions and defenses that may surface and interfere with the best of humanistic medicine.

There are numerous ways to alleviate pain. Recognition of possible depression is essential. Treatment of this condition is best effected by the combined use of antidepressants and psychotherapy. Extremely anxious patients are often best helped by increased contacts with hospital personnel: dieticians, occupational therapists, social service workers, and the like, as well as by the adjuvant use of tranquilizers.

When, in response to their increasing dependency, patients regress and become withdrawn, demanding, or generally difficult, it is important for the helpers to recognize that the patients are not reacting to them personally. Other patients may use their illness to punish or rebel against their families and helpers by misinterpreting instructions, refusing or misusing medications. Health professionals must not be afraid to respond firmly but gently.

In their contacts with the families of patients with cancer, the physicians' role is to steer them away from the extremes of avoidance or excessive closeness to the patient, toward some middle ground. If this is achieved, families can be of great support to patients, who subsequently feel neither abandoned or unloved, nor overwhelmed. Family members benefit, too, since being helpful during this period can assuage future guilt feelings.

One of the most trying tasks for physicians, both at the time of the initial diagnosis and continually afterward, is dealing with the matter of denial. This subject has evolved as an ongoing and ponderous debate over whether "to tell or not to tell." Endless discussions and pages of print have been devoted to the topic. Armed with stockpiles of statistics to support their claims, the defenders of the two opposing positions present compelling arguments. Although the debate is interesting, the question is, in fact, academic. That the question is indeed academic is buttressed by the current era of "informed consent." If physicians tell their patients the awesome truth, they enter a period of shock, but later slip back into denial. If, on the other hand, the decision is made not to divulge the diagnosis or to obfuscate it, somehow the patients know anyway, and do what they have to do (e.g., make financial arrangements, etc.). As mentioned earlier, patients do not permanently surrender this defense, regardless of what physicians say or studiously avoid saying to them.

The best example of this point is the case of a surgeon who believed that patients should be told, quite directly, and trained his residents in this approach. He later developed a carcinoma and his own surgeon, who was one of his former residents, being very well trained, told him "the facts." "Dr. W., you have a carcinoma of...and this is it. You had better make your arrangements." Dr. W. remained in the hospital for a year and almost every day, if he had the chance, tried to have the former resident thrown off the staff.

Denial is *hope*, and as such is as important to cancer patients as are the narcotics they need for pain. The discoveries of insulin and polio vaccine are two examples that bear testimony to the reality of hope. Hope is realistic, too, since no one can predict when a patient will die. Patients constantly outlive predictions about the amount of time they have left, and in some cases, have been known to outlive their doctors as well. A useful technique is to treat patients with cancer as sick but not dying. In a sense this is participation in their denial, a denial that equates with hope. It is not helpful to allow the patient to indulge in self-pity or in lying around waiting to die. This approach often needs to be verbalized in a rather strong manner. Experience shows that patients do mobilize themselves and can be helped to view themselves as "living alongside" of cancer rather than "living with" cancer. In other words, the patient living with cancer implies fighting cancer 24 hours a day. With the attitude of living alongside of cancer, patients find that they can ignore the diagnosis most of the time and think of it only when they are symptomatic.

For physicians, the appropriate question is not *if* but *how* to tell. The key factors are that the telling must be done in a private setting with compassion and with an awareness of timing and the patient's and physician's personalities. Most important, physicians must somehow balance denial with reality, since too much of either is neither necessary nor helpful. If physicians attack their patients' denial too fiercely, they rob them of hope and the patients feel abandoned. If they push too hard on avoidance, however, patients may feel inadequate to cope with the demands that the disease and death pose. Thus, physicians must steer a delicate course between the two, skillfully offering them enough reality while at the same time permitting them the integrity of their denial. Also, physicians must recognize that they unwittingly deny their patients hope (which is their only defense) when they avoid or reject them, or discredit their demands which are only barely disguised pleas for attention.

In terms of treatment, once the matter of telling has been dealt with, the question then becomes what can be done for the patient? Here again, it is a matter of *how* in addition to *what*. Physicians should approach their patients with kindness and hope, leaving grief, futility, and anguish for the family. The modes of therapy and their purposes must be carefully explained to the patient in a clear, unhurried, and supportive manner. It should not be assumed that the patient is knowledgeable about medical procedures even when he happens to be a physician. The experiences of a doctor undergoing therapy for a lymphoma dramatically illustrates the universal requirement for explanation.[9] On the other hand, the treating physician should not be patronizing when a sophisticated patient questions the details of therapy. It is important to permit and indeed encourage patients to retain some measure of control by offering them alternate choices of therapy whenever possible. Active involvement of a patient in his treatment can prevent regression and improve compliance with medical treatment. The language of oncology is often confusing and frightening to the patient.[10] When medical abbreviations and acronyms are discussed in the presence of the patient, they are perceived as a foreign language and often provoke anger and frustration. The cavalier use of terms such as "citrovorum rescue" can produce panic in the most phlegmatic of individuals.[11] There comes a time when the efficacy of further painful or harrowing therapy is doubtful.[12] Physicians then must face the difficult but essential task of relating this to the patient and should allow the dying person the choice of refusing further active treatment. The physician's obligation to relieve pain, alleviate discomfort, and most important to allay anxiety does not cease when the patient refuses to continue with specific treatment.

The most important function physicians can perform during this period is giving patients the opportunity to talk. In the absence of cure, the real art of medicine is in amelioration. This can be achieved by actively listening, not gratuitously offering psychological or religious explanation. Listening is an art, which can be time-consuming, tedious, and emotionally wearing, particularly as one sees one's powers to cure failing, but, nonetheless, can be extremely gratifying. When physicians manage to sublimate their need for omnipotence, the rewards are as great as for the surgeons who successfully perform a difficult operation or for internists who

nurse a coronary through the night. Listening enables
patients to air their fears about life, death, the family,
work, or anything. The "involved" physician permits
his patients to talk freely and openly about very private
matters. In this way, despite the absence of a cure, the
patient's suffering is lessened. This is "art" of medicine
in its ultimate sense. It also allows physicians to
"hear" what their patients are really asking so they
can guide them accordingly. Such guidance is best provided in the form of short, simple statements addressed
to what the patient is saying or asking, not steering
him to another, less charged topic. What is *really* being
asked requires an answer and it must be direct.

Physicians of necessity go through training that
emphasizes the medical-biological model of and for
death. Recently there has evolved a popular, intellectu-
alized philosophical-social-psychological model. Both
are necessary for understanding of dying, grieving,
and gaining insight into one's own feelings. But those
who are experiencing losing and loss need ordinary,
calm, unangry, unfrightened human contact, not par-
rotlike platitudes.

Of what service can the oncologist be in the ending
period? A great deal. The listening continues and at the
very end, the doctor offers sadness as well as hope. Not
tears, for they belong to the family, but the nonverbal
sadness one friend feels for the other on parting. Nor
does the doctor bring hope in the religious sense,
though where it seems appropriate, the physician may
help patients accept a religious death without exerting
his own convictions. The hope to be inferred here is
concerned with self-dignity, achieved by working
through the difficult process of dying, just as one feels a
sense of accomplishment by working through the
equally difficult process of living.

References

1. Schnaper, N. Emotional responses of the surgical patient. In *Tice's Practise of Medicine.*Hagerstown, Maryland; Harper & Row, Vol. X, Chapter 44, 1969, pp. 1-14.

2. Abrams, R.D., and Finesinger, J.E. Guilt reactions in patients with cancer. *Cancer* 6: 474, 1953.

3. Finesinger, J.E., Shands, H.C., and Abrams, R.D. Managing the emotional problems of the cancer patient. In *Clinical Problems in Cancer Research.* Sloan-Kettering Institute Seminar, 1948-1949, American Cancer Society, Inc., 1952, p. 106.

4. Pattison, E.M. Experience of dying. *Am. J. Psychother.* 21: 32, 1967.

5. Schnaper, N. *What* preanesthetic visit? *Anesthesiology 22: 486, 1961.*

6. Schnaper, N. Should an adopted child be told that he is adopted? *Md. State Med. J.* 13: 34, 1964.

7. Schnaper, N. Management of the terminally ill patient and his family. In: *The Psychiatric Foundations of Medicine: Psychiatric Problems in Medical Practice.* Eds. Balis, G.U., Wurmser, L., McDaniel, E. and Grenell, R.G. Boston; Butterworth Publishers Inc. 1978, pp. 231-251.

8. Schnaper, N. Death and dying: Has the topic been beaten to death? *J. Nerv. Ment. Dis.* 160: 3, 1975.

9. Cohn, K. H. Chemotherapy from an insider's perspective. Personal Paper. *Lancet* 1: 1006-1009, 1982.

10. Christy, N.P. English is our second language. Sounding Board. *N. Engl. J. Med.* 300: 979-981, 1979.

11. Schnaper, N. Down the tube? No: Rescue—The language of oncology. *N. Engl. J. Med.* 296: 883, 1977.

12. Schnaper, L.A., Schnaper, N., Fierce, A.R., and Schnaper, H.W. Euthanasia: An overview. *Md. State Med. J.* 26: 42-50, 1977.

THE HOSPICE CONCEPT

Iris Kozil

The term "hospice" derives from a medieval word for a place of shelter for travelers on difficult journeys. The current use of the term defines programs designed to control and relieve the emotional and physical suffering of the terminally ill. This concept originated in Britain, where many hospices have been established during the last 10 years, most notably, St. Christopher's Hospice.

A hospice is a program of medical health care for the terminally ill with very specific, recognizable elements (Table 1).[1] It is an autonomous, centrally administered program of coordinated in- and outpatient services. This physician-directed health care delivery system employs a multifaceted approach in which an interdisciplinary hospice team undertakes to provide psychologic, sociologic, and spiritual services as they are

TABLE 1
BASIC CHARACTERISTICS OF A HOSPICE
PROGRAM

A. The Hospice Program:

Autonomous.
Centrally administered.
A program of coordinated out- and inpatient services, primarily concerned with home care, with back-up inpatient services when home care is not feasible.

B. Primary Unit of Care—Patient and Family:

Total patient care includes dealing with family and other significant patient relationships.

C. Symptom Control:

Physical: pain, nausea, vomiting, and other symptoms are controlled as effectively as medically possible.
Emotional: behavioral sciences are important in helping patient and family cope with emotional distress accompanying impending death.
Spiritual: attention to human spiritual concerns is equally as important as pain care and is integral to a hospice program.

D. Physician-Directed Interdisciplinary Care:

All health care is provided under the direction of a qualified physician.
The interdisciplinary areas include: social work; physical, occupational, and speech therapy; pastoral care, and a wide variety of consultant services (e.g., psychiatric, radiologic, pediatric, oncologic).

E. Trained Volunteers:

Volunteers are specially selected and extensively trained; they augment staff services and are not engaged in lieu of staff.

Volunteers provide vital services other than clinical (e.g., transportation, companionship, recreational and other services).

F. Services Available ON CALL:

Hospice services are available on 7-day a week, 24-hour basis.

Hospice nursing staff bear primary responsibility and call on other program resources as necessary.

G. Staff Support and Communication:

Opportunities for staff to discuss their concerns—either one-to-one, or in a group, on a structured or unstructured basis—are imperative.

Channels for staff discussion, support and mutual evaluation are established.

H. Bereavement Follow-up:

Hospice services are extended to the family during the period of bereavement. Extent and length of bereavement care is based on factors prior to and following death of patient.

I. Hospice Services Based on Need:

Hospice services are based on need rather than ability to pay.

needed. The patient *and* family is the primary unit of
care and services are available on a 24-hour, 7-day-a-
week basis. Patients are usually accepted on the basis
of health needs, rather than ability to pay. Narcotic
and non-narcotic analgesics are used in physical
symptom control. The hospice team will continue support to the bereaved family during the period of
mourning.

The Patient and Family—The Primary Unit of Care

With the great advances made in the diagnosis and
treatment of disease, one can inadvertently lose sight
of the patient; a patient is not merely a collection of
symptoms, but a human being and a member of a
family.[2]

The psychological and social problems that confront
both the terminally ill patient and the patient's family
are often more distressing than the disease itself.
Patients have extremely urgent and practical concerns. Questions often asked are, "How long will it be?"
"How hard is it on my family?" "Will the money last?"[2]

Depression, anxiety, and tension plague the relatives
of the terminally ill as well as the patient. Unfinished
business, a family facing problems of financial support, long-term plans and dreams destroyed by terminal illness—all are legitimate sources of apprehension
and emotional stress. Family members also have many
questions: "How much does he know?" "What should I
tell the children?" "What do I do if there is bleeding in
the middle of the night?" "How will I manage alone?"
These concerns, as well as relief of physical symptoms,
must be met by treatment plans.[2]

Patient/family care generally begins with a visit by a member of the hospice team to the home. In an effort to relate to the patient/family under conditions of stress, it is essential to develop some understanding of their situation: (1) is the patient the sole support of the family? (2) what are the cultural and behavioral family patterns? (3) are there any long-term conflicts or tension in the family situation?

The demands imposed on the family caring for a terminally ill person often cause family members to deny their own needs. This can lead to feelings of neglect and resentment. Unlike acute illness, where recovery is expected, with terminal illness every family member is affected. The hospice team is attentive to the needs of family members as well as to those of the patient. Active participation by family members is encouraged since it has been observed clinically that those who are involved in the care of a loved one are less prone to later develop guilt and self-criticism.

Interdisciplinary Care

The terminally ill are best served by a medical team with a holistic approach to patient care. The typical hospice team includes social work, occupational, physical and speech therapy, pastoral care, and a variety of consultant services (e.g., psychiatric, radiologic, pediatric).

These services are directly supervised by a physician. Patients and their families frequently complain that, in the final stages of terminal illness, they feel abandoned by their physicians. When life-saving measures are no longer available, many physicians, for a number of reasons, feel that their role is at an end and withdraw from the patient. This is not true in the hospice setting where physicians are actively involved at all times.

Symptom Control

One of the major goals of a hospice program is to maintain a reasonable quality of life for the patient. The control of physical and psychological pain is therefore of crucial importance.

Before any regimen can be recommended, a thorough assessment of the physical pain is vital and should include:

- Delineation of site(s): Is it localized, diffuse, referred?
- Does certain activity alleviate or exacerbate pain?
- How is the sleep pattern affected?
- Is the patient taking other medication?[2]

Often, if sufficient information is elicited from the patient, the need for narcotic analgesics may be reduced or other methods can be utilized which could prove to be equally beneficial.

Pharmacologic agents can be effectively used for the palliation of pain. However, inordinate concern regarding the use of powerful narcotics can be an impediment to the care of the terminally ill. Before a successful pharmacologic program of pain relief can be instituted, fears of addiction must be addressed. Physical dependence is not a problem in the patient with terminal cancer, psychological addiction is rare, and tolerance does not pose a clinical problem.[2] Twycross has noted that much of our information about narcotics comes from animal studies, ex-drug addicts, or from patients with acute pain who are usually given single doses parenterally and that application of these findings to patients with chronic pain is questionable. Twycross's studies suggest that common beliefs about long-term use of narcotics may be nothing more than "folklore."[3]

Narcotics are used to relieve severe physical pain when non-narcotic medication or other measures (e.g., spinal block or traction) have failed to control the pain.[3] Hospice regimen combines narcotics with phenothiazines, usually Compazine or prochlorperazine, and these are administered orally. Phenothiazines potentiate the action of the narcotic, thus allowing a lower dose of narcotic. They are antiemetic and will also control anxiety related to chronic pain. Other anxiolytic drugs can be used either in combination with a phenothiazine or, rarely, alone with narcotics.[3]

Patients should not have to wait until pain appears before medication is administered, and the medication can be titrated for each patient's needs.[4] In cancer patients, pain can be unrelenting and overwhelmingly severe. Anxiety and depression are part of the nature of that pain. Fear of the return of the pain induces anxiety which increases the pain. The depression associated with chronic pain may be treated with tricyclic antidepressants (e.g., Elavil). Careful evaluation is crucial since depression may be an entirely appropriate response on the part of the patient and not require medication at all. However, if depression is a contributing factor, the addition of antidepressants can be useful in controlling pain.[3] Perhaps the most innovative aspect of the hospice program is its method of delivering pain medication to patients. Generally, these drugs are self-administered by either the patient or family members.[4] The intention here is to free the patient from dependence upon staff for pain relief and to allow the patient to assume responsibility for the control of his or her pain. For this reason oral doses of narcotic analgesic drugs are preferred because they provide the patient with greater latitude. It has been the hospice experience that pain is much easier to *prevent* than it is to ameliorate after it has made its appearance.

Symptom control involves more than the administration of medication. An environment that is peaceful and secure, providing quality professional care and family interaction—all play a role in the relief of pain. Human spiritual concerns must also be addressed. The guidance and input from pastors of the various religions are integral to the hospice concept.

The Role of Nursing in Hospice Care

The primary responsibility for daily patient care in a hospice setting is in the hands of nurses as they work at the bedside of the dying. It is up to the nurse to ensure patient comfort: wet bed sheets, constipation, and insomnia are practical concerns of critical importance.[5] Quality nursing care entails:[6]

- Imaginative care, unhurried, with attention to detail.
- Learning to perform tasks (e.g., feeding a patient) with patience and devotion, not with a mind on other matters.
- Learning the patient's mode of communication (e.g, understanding the person who cannot speak or does so with great difficulty).
- Learning to sit quietly with the dying, to keep them in touch with life as much as possible, with continuous caring until the end.

• Involvement with the family members after the patient's death, to help in the process of grief.

Staff Support and Communication

Proper patient care of necessity entails "involvement" on the part of professional staff. Intense, interpersonal relationships develop between patients and hospice personnel. Opportunities for staff members to discuss their own feelings are essential. This may be structured or unstructured, on a one-to-one basis or within group meetings. Evaluation and expression of normal and appropriate emotional responses to human sorrow are integral to a hospice program.[7]

Bereavement

In keeping with the concept of the patient *and* family as the unit of care, hospice programs provide professional services during the period of mourning for the surviving family members. Since the grieving are more susceptible to psychological and physical illness, professional medical care for them is entirely logical. Some family members, experiencing a sense of relief after the death of a relative, can become guilt-ridden. Professional care may help resolve this difficulty. Also, the ability to communicate often eases emotional burdens, and hospice professionals can help to initiate or guide this important process. All involved must accept the fact of death and let life go; yet there is a continuity spoken of in all human thought systems that remains and helps the living to go on. These are extremely individual matters and require careful consideration by the hospice team in order to help the family find their own answers.[8]

Volunteers

In most hospice programs throughout the country, trained volunteers play a most significant role. By virtue of their status as non-professionals, volunteers are sometimes in a better position to offer support than are other members of the team. They serve from a perspective beyond the illness. The volunteer is often seen by the patient and family as someone outside the health-care delivery system with whom they are sometimes willing to share thoughts and feelings they would not share with members of the team. Freedom from professional responsibility often permits volunteers to listen and talk at a critical time when the patient is being open and receptive. They can then alert the appropriate professional to the needs of the patient. In home care they can perform all chores that would be assigned to a lay caregiver such as cleaning up and bathing, back rubs, and changing the beds, all of which can improve a patient's overall comfort.

Health Care Needs vs. Ability to Pay

It is the aim of the hospice program to provide medical services on the basis of health needs and not on the ability to pay. Until most recently, hospice programs were dependent upon grants, either public or private, and donations. In September of 1982, the Federal Government passed legislation which will make reimbursement for hospice care part of the Medicare payment plan. This plan will remain in effect for three years with the express purpose of evaluation whether hospice care is less expensive than care provided in acute care hospitals. Many private insurance companies are also taking a careful look at hospice care in order to establish priorities in their reimbursement systems. Standards and certification processes have to be established to make it possible to integrate hospice into the national health care system.

The hospice program is a humane, holistic approach to medical care that has support among all elements of society. Every effort must be made to protect this innovation from profiteering, commercial exploitation, and the lowering of standards and supervision.

References

1. Lack, S.A. Philosophy and organization of a hospice program. Hospice, Inc. reprint.

2. Craven, J., and Wald, F.S. Hospice care for dying patients. *Am. J. Nursing* 75: 1816-1822, 1975.

3. Twycross, R. Clinical experience with diamorphine in advanced malignant disease. *Int. J. Clin. Pharmacol.* 7:198, 1974.

4. Lack, S.A. I want to die while I'm still alive. Paper presented at Conf. on Death and Dying: Education, Counseling and Care, 1976.

5. Dunn, M.D. A philosophy for living (The Hospice Program of Care). Proc. ACS 2nd Natl. Conf. on Cancer Nursing, pp. 95-97, 1977.

6. Galton, V.A. Cancer nursing at St. Christopher's hospice. Proc. of Natl. Conf. on Cancer Nursing, pp. 122-123, 1974.

7. Dobihal, E.F., Jr. Talk on terminal care? *Conn. Med.* 38:364-367, 1974.

8. Craven and Wald, op. cit.

THE MANAGEMENT OF INTRACTABLE PAIN

John M. Merrill

As this book demonstrates, there are many facets to the ordeal of "incurable illness." The specter of intractable pain is a grim one, a curse to anyone, patient or physician, who might dare to say in desperation, "Things just can't get any worse." There is a double tragedy in situations of intractable pain—the suffering of the victim and the ignorance which may allow a poorly managed situation to persist. For it is the premise of this chapter that contemporary pain management makes truly "intractable pain" an infrequent sequela of incurable disease.

We will consider intractable pain which may arise in any pathologic condition, although it is with cancer that intractable pain, or at least the fear of intractable pain, is generally linked. However, cancer is often (for up to half the patients) curable, so no chronic pain need arise. Further, even when incurable, cancer does not invariably cause intractable pain. This prevalent misconception, shared by patients and physicians, compounds the pain problem. As will be seen in the following pages, "chronic pain" differs from "acute pain." Chronic pain is the most deleterious aspect of the cancer/pain myth. Recent research has provided guidelines for estimating when cancer is likely to result in a major pain problem. Daut and Cleeland[1] found that data on the severity, incidence, and pathophysiology of pain with cancer are rare, despite the increased attention given to pain management in both the lay and professional literature. The likelihood of pain varied greatly depending upon the primary site, presence of metastases, and progression of disease. Tumors primary or metastatic to the skeletal system clearly have a potential for considerable pain. Visceral tumors, primary or secondary, are often painless. The experienced clinician can anticipate when a cancer pain problem is likely to occur. Expectant management is preferable, easier, and more humane than having to treat severe established pain.

Acute and Chronic Pain

Acute pain has been termed "linear"—having a defined beginning, and is expected by the patient and physician to have a defined and generally proximate end. One rarely encounters intractable acute pain or even hears such a description. There is the tacit assumption that acute pain is usually a short-term problem adequately managed with whatever analgesic is necessary.

Chronic pain has been referred to as "circular" pain, which carries the recollection of previously experienced pain and a certain expectation of a painful future. The patient with a chronic and painful condition has an emotional reaction to the pain, usually fear and an absolute dread of its recurrence and persistence. Accompanying anxiety and depression, so common in the chronically ill, will also serve to intensify the pain.

Reuler et al.,[2] in a recent comprehensive review on pain management, state, "The management of chronic pain is a universal and vexing problem for physicians." This review documents the poor understanding many health professionals have of basic concepts relating to pain. Such ignorance generally assumes that the physician will be frustrated and the patient inadequately relieved.

It behooves every physician to become well-informed of pharmacologic and technologic advances in the area of pain management so that he is equipped with the most up-to-date armamentarium. Yet, these advances alone cannot be allowed to defocus the humanistic approach to caring for the patient with pain.

Problems of Tolerance and Addiction

I will cite one area of misunderstanding of the pharmacology of analgesic drugs and emphasize what the human factor of the doctor-patient relationship must contribute to the pursuit of satisfactory pain relief. The issue is that of "pharmacologic tolerance." "Tolerance" may be confused with "addiction." Tolerance is the change in response of any physiologic system of the body to the same dose of medication over time. There is generally a reduced response over time—which may take weeks or months. Addiction is that state of physical and mental dependence upon a drug in which specific body disturbances follow with withdrawal of the agent. There is often a behavioral pattern of compulsive drug abuse in the addicted patient. Addiction in cancer patients without a previous history of drug abuse or alcoholism is rare and may take months to develop, if ever.

Pharmacologic tolerance, however, is common, and the experienced clinician not only expects it but can use the phenomenon to ease the patient through the initial days of a program to combat chronic pain.

Narcotic analgesics, virtually always needed eventually for the chronic pain of an incurable affliction, have a sedative side-effect. Tolerance to this usually develops within days, and the patient and family can be reassured that somnolence will shortly be decreased but may be a therapeutic adjunct in the first days of a challenging pain problem. Tolerance to the euphoria induced by narcotics develops most rapidly. This leads to the compulsive drug-seeking which characterizes drug abusers when euphoria is the goal of drug use. For the pain patient, however, analgesia is the goal, and fortunately, tolerance to this effect takes weeks to months to develop.

While the "street addict" rapidly escalates drug dosages, the pain patient's need for increased dose is generally found to relate to disease progression.[3] The common side-effect of decreased gastrointestinal motility secondary to narcotics can cause severe discomfort, so precautions against obstipation must be maintained. Narcotics may depress the respiratory drive. However, pain is a strong respiratory stimulus as well, and generally, respiratory depression is not a problem that interferes with achieving adequate analgesic levels. Thus "tolerance" is a multifaceted phenomenon in the pain-management setting.

Administration of Chronic Analgesics

The "PRN" ("pro re nata," according to circumstances) administration of analgesics is appropriate for acute pain. There is an expectation that the need for such medication, both dose and frequency, will be reduced in a short time. Chronic pain, however, generally demands regular dosage intervals. It takes a smaller dose to prevent pain than to treat it. The use of a regimen of PRN doses in patients with chronic pain promotes drug-seeking behavior and probably has a greater addicting potential, based on behavioral modification models. Chronic pain control demands that a dose adequate for substantial relief be found, then given regularly. Most patients with chronic pain will accept some degree of residual pain. Once a level of comfort is assured, the patient is free to contend with the other aspects of the chronic disease state. The regular administration of analgesics tends to diminish whatever adversarial problem may arise among the patients, their families, and the professional staff.

New Developments in Pain Pathophysiology

Recent discoveries in the biochemistry of pain modulation have shown that the body, specifically areas of the central nervous system, produces its own endogenous opiates known as "endorphins." Though beyond the scope of this chapter, these substances are 20-30 times more potent than morphine and may be the analgesics of the future. How these substances are elaborated or what functions are involved is under intense study.[4] The substances may explain the response to such pain relief methods as acupuncture and percutaneous nerve stimulators for pain control.

Better neuroanatomical knowledge may lead to precise ablative procedures when destruction of the actual route of the pain response is indicated.[5]

Analgesic Adjuncts

Aspirin and the narcotic agents are the basic pharmacologic preparations for analgesia. There are other agents which can be adjunctive, including the psychoactive drugs such as phenothiazines and tricyclics. "Pain cocktails" are in vogue, e.g., Brompton's Mixture. Although the pioneering hospice work with narcotics often included several ingredients besides the opiates (e.g., cocaine), more recent research has demonstrated that the narcotics alone are the effective analgesic ingredient.[6]

Consumerism/Humanism in Pain Management

The experienced, compassionate physician welcomes the participation of the patient in the efforts to control pain. The patient should expect his physician to be knowledgeable about pain or willing to consult experts. Many institutions now have multi-disciplinary pain teams whose members may include neurosurgeons, anesthesiologists, psychiatrists, pharmacologists, oncologists, physical therapists, nurses, and other health care professionals. This team paradigm for pain control is not always needed, but the concern of the physician for his patient is. The humanism demonstrated in patient care is a crucial adjunct to the drug prescribed.

More recently, the physician can expect a better-informed "consumer." The humanistic health-care provider is not threatened by the informed lay person, and there are improved resources for the lay public including a newly released, free monograph on pain control from the National Cancer Institute, published by the American Cancer Society.[7]

In conclusion, it may be assumed that pain resulting from tissue injury will remain a frequently encountered management problem for the indefinite future. However, ignorance about its control can be eliminated. In the context of the incurable patient, the relief of pain may be the best response to the French folk admonition: "To cure sometimes, to relieve often, to comfort always."

References

1. Daut, R.L., Cleeland, C.S. The prevalance and severity of pain in cancer. *Cancer* 50:1913-1918, 1982.

2. Reuler, J.B., Girard, D.E., Nardone, D.A. The chronic pain syndrome: misconceptions and management. *Ann. Intern. Med.* 93:588-596, 1980.

3. Marks, R.M., Sachar, E.J. Undertreatment of medical-inpatients with narcotic analgesics. *Ann. Intern. Med.* 78:173-181, 1973.

4. Goodman, C.E. Pathophysiology of pain. *Arch. Intern. Med.* 143:527-530, 1983.

5. Brechner, V.L., Ferrer-Brechner, T., Allen G.D. Anes-

thetic measures in management of pain associated with malignancy. *Sem. Oncology* 4:99-108, 1977.

6. Melzack, R., Mount, B.M., Gordon, J.M. The Brompton Mixture versus morphine solution given orally: effects on pain. *Can. Med. Assoc. J.* 120:435-438, 1979.

7. National Cancer Institute Publication. *Questions and Answers about Pain Control*, American Cancer Society, New York, 1983.

THE PHYSICIAN'S ATTITUDE TOWARD MENTAL ILLNESS

Marc H. Hollender

For several decades, psychiatrists have made a concerted effort to alter the attitude of other physicians toward mental illness, in particular, the attitude toward somatizing disorders and emotional disturbances secondary to physical illness. To this end, consultation-liaison psychiatrists have participated in patient care on medical and surgical services, and other psychiatrists have conducted clinical exercises and taught regular and special courses.

The premise was that, with more effective teaching, a new generation of physicians would approach patients differently than their predecessors. Everyday observations and anecdotal reports, however, indicate that the attitude of many—perhaps most—physicians toward mental illness still carries a negative valence. Reports based on the responses of physicians to questionnaires bear this out.[1,2,3] So, too, do the findings of studies on

117

the resistance of physicians to requesting psychiatric consultations.[4,5] However, a somewhat more positive note about the physician's attitude toward mental illness has appeared in the literature recently.[6,7]

Although these surveys suggest that the attitude of physicians toward emotional disturbances may be somewhat more favorable than it was in years past, the question still must be posed: Is it really more favorable or does it merely seem to be? Are we taken in by lip service? Has the negative attitude, like outspoken prejudice, simply gone underground?

For our present purpose, the assumption will be made that, although there is considerable individual variation among physicians and some indications of a generally more positive approach, the prevailing overall attitude toward emotional disturbances is much less accepting than would be optimal for good patient care. The focus of this chapter will be on the forces that shape the physician's reactions and coping mechanisms.

Physical and Mental Illness: Same or Different

A few decades ago, an attempt was made in some quarters to whitewash mental illness by declaring that it was the same as physical illness. As might have been anticipated, this approach proved as unsuccessful as the attempt to make the latter years of life more palatable by labeling them the "golden age." Fundamental differences do exist, and no whitewash job will ever obliterate them.

The kind of pitfall created when an effort is made to declare that physical and mental illnesses are the same is clearly seen in the following instance. In writing about confidentiality, Sieglar stated, "The keeping of separate psychiatric records implies that psychiatry and medicine are different undertakings and thus drives deeper the wedge between them and between physical and psychological illnesses."[8]

Certainly, to release information about a gall-bladder operation is distinctly and sometimes drastically different than releasing information about a marital conflict or a sexual problem—and undoubtedly always will be. The hard fact is that to a considerable extent "psychiatry and medicine are different undertakings," and the wedge between them will not be removed by declaring them to be the same. A more reasonable and productive approach might be to broaden the base so that differences can be accommodated.

Broadening the Base: The Biopsychosocial Model

In recent years, the need for a holistic approach to patient care has been emphasized.[9] Still, the model underlying much of current medical practice is biological rather than biopsychosocial. Physicians generally prefer to regard the human body as a machine and take steps to repair defects or correct dysfunctions. Certainly, such an approach circumscribes and simplifies their task. As Pilowsky stated, "If the natural history of an illness were dependent for its characteristics only upon the nature of the pathological changes which underlay it, doctors would experience a professional existence of remarkable simplicity and predictability."[10]

Essentially, the same thesis was expressed with a touch of levity in the following statement: "Unfortunately, the patient's personality tends to interfere with the wonderful relationship the doctor could have with the disease."[11]

In addressing the same issue, Bennet stated, "There is unfortunately a certain amount of evidence that many doctors simply do not want to know about the patient as a person; they would, on the whole, prefer it if they could study and treat the pathological process in, say, the heart or the liver without having to have those organs lodged in a human frame."[12]

Bennet cited as an example the case of a patient complaining of indigestion. The physician evinced interest when told the pain came on two to three hours after meals but showed no interest when the patient mentioned her son's impending appearance in court. Bennet concluded, "When the doctor disregards the lady's remarks about her son's impending appearance in court it is either because he believes such details to be irrelevant or else because he does not know what to do with them or how to evaluate them."

In a study on possible emotional antecedents of bleeding from peptic ulcer[13], it was noted that 7 of 15 patients had been confronted one to three days prior to bleeding by conflict situations that they could not resolve and that resulted in intense feelings of frustration, helplessness, or despair. Such information is not likely to be elicited if the physician restricts the focus to physical symptoms whether by failing to inquire about emotional antecedents or by discouraging the expression of them.

The following case note is an example. For a 49-year-old man, the precipitating event seemed to be his mistress's threat that, if he did not leave his wife to marry her, she would accept the proposal of another man. The patient struggled with the ultimatum but decided not to leave his wife. Although he had been impotent with her for several years, he felt she was a "good woman," and he was deeply attached to her. During his last meeting with his mistress, he told her of his decision. His bleeding began the next day. During the period in which he was making the decision, he experienced "hunger pains" relieved by food or milk.

Only by broadening the base to include psychosocial factors is it possible to understand some illnesses. Even physicians who agree with this statement are likely to regard psychological disturbances as unwanted and annoying complications. How physicians will react, however, will depend on their preparation intellectually and emotionally to cope with mental illnesses in their patients.

Medical School Education: Its Effect on Attitude

In spite of improvements in medical school courses in psychiatry—they have come a long way since an alienist would present two or three lectures on the psychoses—for many physicians psychiatry remains relatively foreign and unfamiliar territory. Several studies bear out this contention.

Greenbank, in a study of the graduates of the five medical schools in Philadelphia, found serious deficiencies in knowledge.[14] For example, one-half of the respondents thought that a person who talks of suicide hardly ever carries out the act, and one-half thought that mental illness is frequently caused by masturbation.

Castelnuovo-Tedesco assessed how much psychiatry medical students learn using the responses to a questionnaire of 110 interns, residents, and fellows representing a cross section of American and Canadian schools.[15] Over one-third stated that their training was indifferent or poor, and one-half believed that they had not learned as much about psychiatry as they would need to practice medicine. Twenty percent stated that they would try to avoid neurotic patients, and 16% would not want to spend more time, even if available, discussing the personal problems of their patients.

In a study of 219 young Navy physicians from 70 medical schools, Tucker and Reinhardt found that those physicians with favorable attitudes toward psychiatry had significantly more exposure to psychiatry courses in medical school.[16]

Additional information about physicians' knowledge of and attitude toward mental illness was gathered from a survey of their reactions to suicide. Rockwell and O'Brien found that 27% of physicians (non-psychiatrists) would feel uncomfortable talking with patients about suicide.[17] Only 54% would accept into their practices without hesitancy persons who previously attempted suicide. The authors concluded: "Physicians have some significant gaps in knowledge about and attitudes toward suicide that interfere with their being as effective in suicide prevention as they might be."

Any situation for which preparation is inadequate is likely to engender feelings that are disquieting. A feeling of incompetency may spark off anxiety and guilt. Various mechanisms then can be used to avoid or fend off discomfort. Stoller and Geertsma described one particular sequence of events.[18] While in medical school, students become aware of discomfort in dealing with patients with emotional difficulties. In addition to experiencing frustration and irritability, students also suffer from consciously felt guilt because of their inadequacy in understanding and treating these patients. As their education progresses, the appropriate reaction to their inadequacy is too easily and too often replaced by scorn. The replacement of guilt by scorn may be reinforced and even encouraged by the example of teachers who use the same coping strategy.

Although the use of scorn as a defensive maneuver may fend off guilt, a feeling of comfort is bought at too high a price. Students and later practitioners who use scorn tend to judge rather than evaluate, and they may regard patients' disorders not as illnesses but as immoral states for which patients are to blame.

In some medical schools, the courses and clinical experience in psychiatry, even if relatively adequate, hardly counterbalance the teachings in other departments. The educational process still may be oriented much too much toward disease and away from the patient. In addition, Engel deplored the failure of educators to appreciate the difference between compassion as a human quality and the acquisition and application of skills in evaluating and resolving human problems.[19] It should be recognized that compassion in itself is no more likely to cure a depression than it is to cure an acute appendicitis.

The Meaning of Mental Illness

Many physicians accept the prevailing outlook toward mental illness in our culture. In keeping with this outlook, physical illness is usually regarded as a "happening," an impersonal event for which no responsibility is assigned and no stigma is attached. In contrast, mental illness is usually regarded as an "action," a personal event for which responsibility is assigned and stigma is attached.

Mental illness is often equated with weakness, lack of moral fiber, and dependence. An extreme attitude—too extreme even for general acceptance in our culture—is typified by the attitude of General George Patton. It is permissible and acceptable to require care if there is a demonstrable infection or lesion; it is not generally as permissible and acceptable if there is no demonstrable organic process as in anxiety state or depression.

In view of the fact that mental illness involves volition, physicians assume that if patients exert sufficient will power they will be able to overcome their symptoms. The approach of some physicians involves the liberal use of non-medicinal prescriptions (i.e., advice to take a vacation, change jobs, have a baby, etc.). It is assumed that non-medicinal prescriptions have few side-effects and can be handed out with impunity. Unfortunately, such is far from the case.[20]

The following instance illustrates the danger involved in the ill-advised use of a non-medicinal prescription. A young woman consulted an internist for a stabbing pain below her left breast accompanied by a fear of dying that she thought was caused by heart disease. Other symptoms were dizziness often followed by faintness. When physical and laboratory examinations failed to reveal an organic basis for these symptoms, she asked to be referred to a psychiatrist. Her physician rejected this request, maintaining that she did not need psychiatric help. He suggested that she take a vacation.

Instead of following this advice, she consulted a second internist. After examining her, he, too, recommended that she take a vacation. When she asked to be referred to a psychiatrist, this physician confided in her, telling her that he had had symptoms much like hers and that he had overcome them by himself without help. He also said that he would not recommend a referral to a psychiatrist. It was not until she became tearful and stated that she must have help that he reluctantly agreed to refer her. It was learned by the psychiatrist she consulted that she was afraid of losing control and harming her children.

People generally, and physicians are no exceptions, tend to expect others to react as they would or as they anticipate they would react in a given situation. Thus, in the case of the second physician, there was the expectation that the patient would use the approach that had worked for him, that she should take a vacation (no doubt to garner strength), and then use self-determination and exercise control.

Mental illness is sometimes equated with badness or sinfulness in our culture. When such a connection is made, the physician may condemn a patient, and the patient may react by feeling guilty. Because the interchange is sometimes subtle, its real nature may go unrecognized.

Mental Illness and Real Medicine

Physicians often contend that psychiatry is inexact and therefore not a science. Carried one step further, the contention is that psychiatry is not real medicine. This stand may be taken to justify a negative attitude toward patients with emotional disturbance. It leads incidentally to the assumption that a medical education is wasted on future psychiatrists. Consequently, students who declare their intention of becoming psychiatrists may receive considerably less attention from their teachers on medical and surgical services.[21]

The inexactness of other aspects of medicine has not troubled physicians to the extent that the inexactness of psychiatry has troubled them. Perhaps it is not the inexactness but the nature of the subject matter that is really troublesome. Instead of dealing, as does medicine, with how an endocrine system works or an ion pump functions—neat, clean, and mechanical—psychiatry deals with sex, guilt, shame, dependence, aggression, and hostility—unsavory, messy, and personal. In addition, probably lying behind the complaint of inexactness, discomfort is caused by unconscious forces—in physicians as well as in others.

The medical student's attitude about psychiatry as an inexact field and the influence of the teaching program is brought out in the following instance. Scully et al. stated, "When it was made clear to them [medical students] that failure to acquire the necessary knowledge and skills, as well as failure to achieve the attitudinal goals of the teaching program, would result in a failing grade in the course, students reacted with anger and incredulity. They argued that psychiatric knowledge was not 'objective' and could not be measured and that psychiatry was not 'important' enough to warrant a failing grade. Eventually, however, the enforcement of our belief that psychiatry was both objective and important resulted in its being viewed as a more legitimate area of study, the duties and requirements of which were as real as those of any other specialty."[22]

Mental Illness and Psychiatric Referral

In adult medical units at Long Island Jewish-Hillside Medical Center, Steinberg et al. found a psychiatric morbidity of 20.8% and a referral rate of only 2.2%.[23] In more than 50% of the patients not referred, physician resistance was involved. Usually, the physicians believed that there was no psychiatric problem or that psychiatry could not help. Less often, the physicians thought that the patient might become upset or that the patient-doctor relationship would be destroyed. In 26 of 29 patients seen, the physician's resistance was not justified; 23 of these patients were judged to be helped by the psychiatrist.

Steinberg et al. stated, "Sometimes physicians fear that their patients will feel offended, angered, or stigmatized by psychiatric consultation, thus compromising their own relationship with the patients. This fear was shown to be unrealistic in the great majority of cases."[24]

Koran et al. noted that referring physicians frequently were concerned that their patients would feel rejected or be regarded as crazy or as having no real disease.[25] Their study, however, revealed that most general hospital patients referred for psychiatric consultation had a positive attitude toward the referral when properly prepared, and most patients found the consultation helpful.

To balance the picture, however, it must be acknowledged that in some instances the physician's experiences with psychiatric referrals may discourage their use. Such is the case when the psychiatrist does not send back information, avowedly because of a concern about confidentiality, or sends back a report studded with jargon that fails to address issues of immediate concern. The physician's attitude can be expected to be positive only if useful information is supplied or if the psychiatrist helps directly and indicates the reasons for a particular approach and the results that might be achieved.

Often it is assumed that patients with serious medical illnesses "have the right to be depressed." Some dysphoria or depressive reaction may be an appropriate response, but the possibility of a second illness, a major depression, should not be dismissed without carefully weighing the possibility. When the patient's response seems severe or out of proportion, a psychiatric referral is certainly indicated.

The Physician's Personality

Emotional forces within physicians, many of them rooted in the unconscious, exert considerable influence on their attitude toward mental illness. Ford pointed out that patients with problems in regard to interpersonal relationships, dependency, addiction, or somatization have the capacity to tap into physicians' conflicts of a similar nature.[26] To defend against anxiety, physicians may not want to hear about depressive symptoms, dependent needs, or marital problems. Consequently, such considerations may be summarily excluded as irrelevant.

When physicians are confronted by their patient's emotional problems in spite of diversionary efforts, they may employ various mechanisms to fend off or avoid disquieting and disturbing feelings. For example, they may focus on physical complaints and dismiss suggestions that psychosocial factors are pertinent. Or they may deal with the situation by referring the patient to a psychiatrist with the referral being an act of extrusion rather than a positive move. Or they may demand that the patient overcome psychological problems by an act of willpower.

In their statement and by their manner, physicians let patients know what verbalizations they want to hear. Some communications are encouraged or reinforced. For example, statements about symptoms may regularly evoke a response of interest. Conversely, other communications are discouraged or extinguished. For example, statements about emotional reactions may consistently be interrupted by questions about bodily dysfunction. In a short time, most relatively compliant or needful patients will learn "to play the game" according to the implicit or explicit rules that have been set down. As a result, they appear to be "purely medical patients," free of psychological distress.

This situation, which often prevails, serves to protect the physician from uncomfortable feelings. However, a price is paid by patients who cannot turn to their physician at a time of stress for understanding, support, and definitive help. Compassion shown by the physician is important, but, in itself, it is not sufficient.

Educational Goals

Progress that has been made in changing the attitude of physicians toward mental illness can largely be attributed to broadening the scope and enriching the content of the teaching of psychiatry in medical school. Further progress must await direct help to students in dealing with their reactions to seriously ill and emotionally disturbed patients in clinical settings.

The students' identification with the patient is the basis for their understanding of psychological distress, but it may also be the cause of much anxiety and personal discomfort. All too often students retreat and detach themselves; disidentification or dehumanization then replaces identification. When this occurs, patients are treated like pathological (inanimate) specimens (machines) rather than like feeling human beings.

Our objective in working with students in clinical

settings should be to help them move from identification to empathy rather than from identification to dis-identification. Empathy, as used here, refers to an admixture of identification and isolation, with isolation meaning the separation of an idea from its emotional charge. This state produces a compromise between the patient's need for closeness and the physician's need for distance. If this state is achieved, it should be possible to cope with psychological problems without losing the objectivity essential for medical practice.

Our educational goals are clear, but the way to reach them is much less clear. Classroom learning is important, but, in itself, it is not enough. The physician's attitude toward mental illness will carry a positive valence only if the learning process for medical students addresses their emotional as well as their intellectual needs.

References

1. Tucker, G.J., Reinhardt, R.F. Attitudes of young physicians: implications for teaching. *Am. J. Psychiatry* 124: 986-990, 1968.

2. Krakowski, A.J. Psychiatric consultation in the general hospital: an exploration of resistances. *Dis. Nerv. Syst.* 36: 242-244, 1973.

3. Rockwell, D.A., O'Brien, W. Physicians' knowledge and attitudes about suicide. *J.A.M.A.* 225:1347-1349, 1973.

4. Steinberg, H., Torem, M., Saravoy, S.M. An analysis of physician resistance to psychiatric consultations. *Arch. Gen. Psychiatry* 37: 1007-1012, 1980.

5. Koran, L.M., Van Natta, J., Stephens, J.R., Pascualy, R. Patients' reactions to psychiatric consultation. *J.A.M.A.* 241:1603-1605, 1979.

6. Hull, J. Psychiatric referrals in general practice. *Arch. Gen. Psychiatry* 36:406-408, 1979.

7. Fauman, M.A. Psychiatric components of medical and surgical practice: a survey of general hospital physicians. *Am. J. Psychiatry* 138: 1298-1301, 1981.

8. Sieglar, M. Confidentiality in medicine—a decrepit concept. *N. Engl. J. Med.* 307:1518-1521, 1983.

9. Engel, G.L. The need for a new medical model: a challenge for biomedicine. *Science* 196:129-136, 1977.

10. Pilowsky, I. Dimensions of abnormal illness behavior. *Aust. N.Z. J. Psychiatry* 9:141-147, 1975.

11. Detre, Katherine. Personal communication, 1975.

12. Bennet, G. Scientific medicine? *Lancet* 2:453-456, 1974.

13. Hollender, M.H., Soults, F.B., Ringold, A.L. Emotional antecedents of bleeding from peptic ulcer. *Psychiatry Med.* 2:199-204, 1971.

14. Greenbank, R.K. Are medical students learning psychiatry? *Pa. Med. J.* 64:989-992, 1961.

15. Castelnuovo-Tedesco, P. How much psychiatry are medical students really learning? *Arch. Gen. Psychiatry* 16:668-675, 1967.

16. Tucker and Reinhardt, op. cit.

17. Rockwell and O'Brien, op. cit.

18. Stoller, R.J., Geertsma, R.H. Measurements of medical students' acceptance of emotionally ill patients. *J. Med. Educ.* 33: 585-590, 1958.

19. Engel, GL. Care and feeding of the medical student— the foundations for professional competence. *J.A.M.A.* 215:1135-1141, 1971.

20. Hollender, M.H. *Psychology of Medical Practice.* Philadelphia: W.B. Saunders, 1958.

21. Crowder, M.K., Hollender, M.H. The medical student's choice of psychiatry as a career: a survey of one graduating class. *Am. J. Psychiatry* 138:505-508.

22. Scully, J.H., Dubovsky, S.L., Simons, R.C. Undergraduate education and recruitment into psychiatry. *Am. J. Psychiatry* 140:573-576, 1983.

23. Steinberg et al., op. cit.

24. Ibid.

25. Koran et al., op. cit.

26. Ford, C.V. *The Somatizing Disorders-Illness As a Way of Life.* New York: Elsevier Biomedical, 1983.

THE CARE OF THE DEMENTED PATIENT

Charles E. Wells

Humanism as an attitude can be valued only in its application.

Anonymous

Every physician who is worth the name must play at least two (and perhaps more) major roles simultaneously. The first is that of caretaker or even servant to the person who is sick, i.e., to the patient. The second is that of combatant against disease. With two such disparate images to fulfill, it is little wonder that the roles are at times in conflict, that they may appear incompatible, or that one may even have to be abandoned for the other in particular situations. The skillful physician spends a lifetime trying to juggle these two roles, to assure that the one does not win out over the other. The one who serves the sick can never be just that, to the neglect of the one who battles disease. Nor can the latter become a knight errant, always questing for a new disease to conquer to the neglect of the patient's personal and human needs.

With a disorder such as dementia, which in the past has offered so few specific therapeutic opportunities, one might have envisaged a situation that would promote full play for the caring, nurturing sides of the physician. Without weapons to fight disease, the physician might have been expected to put on the mantle of concerned caretaker for the demented person, free, at least in this situation, of the need to balance the two roles. Regrettably, such was not the case. All that we know of the past suggests that demented persons have always been shunned by physicians, responsibility for their care being relegated for the most part to non-professionals, with physicians involving themselves little in either the planning or direction of their treatment and care. If a lesson were to be drawn from such a pattern of behavior, it might be that, if physicians lack tools either to combat disease directly or to alleviate the symptoms of disease specifically, they find it difficult, if not impossible, to play out the role of caretaker effectively and enthusiastically.

So far as the care of the demented is concerned, there have been enormous changes over the past ten to twelve years. These changes probably result, for the most part, from three major factors. First came the recognition that not all dementia is untreatable, or more exactly that dementia can be the result of many diseases, some of which respond to specific therapeutic interventions. This was brought to medical attention first and perhaps most forcefully through the description by Hakin, Adams, and associates[1,2] of the syndrome of occult or normal pressure hydrocephalus, a "treatable" form of dementia. This was followed shortly by the report of Marsden and Harrison[3] of a group of over 100 patients referred to them for thorough medical and neurologic evaluation of their dementia. Among these patients, Marsden and Harrison found several whose dementia resulted from reversible medical disorders, several whose dementia resulted from medical and neurologic disorders which, though not reversible, could nevertheless be modified by treatment, several whose symptoms were the result of functional psychiatric disorders, and several who were not demented at all. These findings were soon replicated in studies from neuropsychiatric centers all over the world. These investigations revealed that if patients with apparent dementia were subjected to thorough medical and neuropsychiatric evaluation, about 10-15 percent would be found whose clinical abnormalities could be reversed by appropriate disease-specific treatment and another 25-30 percent whose clinical course could be modified, if not reversed, by appropriate disease-specific treatment.[4] Dementia was transformed thereby from an untreatable into a potentially treatable clinical phenomenon.

The second important factor in this transformation was the recognition that not every patient who appears to be demented is actually demented. Two follow-up studies from Great Britain[5,6] revealed that it was not unusual for patients diagnosed as having presenile dementia to fail to follow the downhill course expected for these disorders. Some indeed recovered completely without specific treatment, leading to the suspicion that the patient's dysfunction had been due to functional psychiatric disorders rather than due to one of the diseases causing dementia. Experiences such as these led to the concept of pseudodementia—a descriptive term for instances in which dementia was mimicked or caricatured by a variety of functional psychiatric disorders.[7,8]

The third factor changing the way physicians deal

with dementia was the recognition that most dementia is probably due to a specific disorder—Alzheimer's disease[9]—and that it is possible, even without disease-specific diagnostic markers, to diagnose Alzheimer's disease with some accuracy during life.[10]

Thus, within a period of little more than a decade, the concept of dementia was changed from that of an untreatable syndrome due to unknown cause to that of a syndrome for which the etiology can almost always be established and for which disease-specific treatment measures are often effective. This is a field then in which enormous medical progress has been achieved, but almost all the progress has centered on specific disease diagnosis and treatment. A role has been defined then, in the medical care of demented patients, for the physician who would fight disease. The role has yet to be spelled out, though, for the physician who would nurture and care for demented patients even though their dementia be caused by diseases for which no specific treatment is known. Is it not possible, therefore, that all the progress of the past decade has failed to change the way that the vast majority of demented patients—those whose dementia is due to irreversible disorders—are cared for by physicians? Is it not just possible that fifteen years ago demented patients and their families were dismissed by physicians with a statement that no treatment was available for dementia (or for hardening of the arteries, as it was generally called then), whereas now they are dismissed with a statement that no treatment is available for Alzheimer's disease?

If this is the case (and certainly anecdotes affirming it abound), it is unlikely that the human needs of demented patients and of their families are neglected because of any basic crassness or insensitivity on the part of physicians toward these patients. It would appear much more likely that neglect, if it occurs, arises because physicians so often experience intense feelings of impotence when they encounter the patient whose dementia is due to an untreatable disease and whose symptoms do not respond predictably to traditional forms of medical intervention. Stated thusly, the average physician's sense of powerlessness is understandable. How can matters be changed? Is there an approach to the demented patient whereby the physician's sense of impotence can be replaced by a sense of mission in the case of the demented patient?

Such a change is possible, but, for it to take place, a basic readjustment must occur in two attitudes which most physicians probably now hold toward the demented patient. First, physicians must abandon the belief that accurate diagnosis, valuable as it is, is the most important service that they can perform for demented patients. Accurate disease diagnosis is important, and indeed it should be considered a right for every patient, but it is not the "be-all" and "end-all" of medical intervention. In other words, at the present level of their knowledge, physicians must weight their aims more heavily toward the care of the patient and the patient's family and less toward the fight against the specific disease causing the dementia. In this area, medical care must become focused more on patients and less on diseases.

Second, physicians must abandon the idea that the only worthwhile medical intervention for the demented patient must have improved cognitive function as its major objective. Such is an unnecessarily restrictive view of the nature of dementia. Although cognitive changes are paramount in dementia, affective and behavioral changes are often almost equally severe.

Indeed, every aspect of the patient's and the family's life may be devastated by dementia, so that the physician who aims only for cognitive change ignores many treatable and changeable clinical elements of dementia.

In order for physicians to give up these two generally accepted attitudes, however, they must be provided with an alternative approach to the demented patient that offers them some sense of mastery and effectiveness. A "function-oriented" approach to the demented patient offers the physician just such an opportunity. Such a strategy accords to an analysis of function disturbances in dementia an importance equal to the pursuit of disease diagnosis. Specifically, it is suggested that the physician make efforts to answer two key questions in every patient who appears to be demented: (1) What *disturbances in function* are present in the patient, and can they be modified? (2) What *diseases*, if any, affect the patient's brain, and can they be modified by disease-specific treatment measures? Thus, functional assessment assumes an importance equal to disease diagnosis.

What is meant by function assessment in dementia? Essentially, functional assessment requires a thorough and detailed evaluation of every aspect of the patient's medical and neuropsychiatric status—assessment of medical status, assessment of behavior (and especially of problem behaviors), assessment of the patient's capacities to perform the ordinary tasks of daily living, assessment of thought processes, assessment of the affective state, assessment of the environment, assessment of the support system. Such a thoughtful and detailed assessment of function will *always* provide the physician with opportunities for useful intervention. Indeed, such a functional analysis is much more likely to provide the physician guidance in the prescription of therapy for the demented patient than is a limited disease oriented approach.

For example, analysis of the medical status may reveal use of medications that are no longer needed but that may be causing further impairment of brain function. Analysis of behavior may reveal behavioral regression that is out of keeping with the severity of the cognitive loss, and the patient may improve markedly in the functions of daily living through the use of specifically designed behavioral treatment techniques. Careful attention to thought processes may uncover paranoid or other varieties of psychotic thinking which may respond well to small doses of antipsychotic medications. Even though the patient may not appear typically depressed, the history of rapidly progressive cognitive loss along with talk that is perseverative on themes of loss may prompt a diagnosis of depression (superimposed on dementia) which may respond well to conventional antidepressant treatments. Depression arising early in the course of dementia and precipitated by awareness of failing powers also may be helped appreciably by supportive psychotherapy. Analysis of the environment may reveal that the family is unaware of the extent of lost function and accordingly is making inappropriate and excessive demands on the patient and perhaps even blaming the patient for not trying. Improvement may then quickly follow the family's increased awareness and knowledge. Analysis of the family support system may find members of the family profoundly ignorant of the nature of the patient's disorder or guilt-ridden because all their efforts to help come to naught or stressed beyond their human limits trying to satisfy the needs of a severely regressed demented family member. Again, attention to the family and its problems may benefit both patient and family. Such a functional analysis will almost always uncover multiple opportunities for intervention with therapeutic tools that are already available—behavioral, psychotherapeutic, pharmacologic. Only if the physician insists on cognitive improvement will he or she be found powerless.

Opposition to such a functional approach might arise for two reasons. First, such patient evaluations and therapeutic techniques require much time and often involve treatment modalities with which many physicians are unfamiliar or uncomfortable. To a certain extent these objections can be overcome by the use of nonphysician medical personnel (nurse specialists, social workers, occupational and recreational therapists, psychologists) to fulfill specific functions both in the evaluation and treatment and as authority to whom patient and families turn for ultimate decisions.

Second, a treatment approach based on functional assessment will strike some as a retreat from recent scientific advances in the diagnosis and treatment of dementia, even perhaps a retreat from the medical model. It must be emphasized that the suggestion that physicians pay more attention to functional assessment and treatment in no way implies that they should pay less attention to the search in the demented patient for specific disease diagnosis and its treatment. Indeed, a functional approach can provide the best medical care possible for the demented patient only if specific disease diagnosis and treatment are assured. Furthermore, a functional approach is by no means foreign to the medical model or foreign to other medical specialties that are firmly entrenched in the medical school. Cardiologists, for example, seldom treat myocardial infarctions directly and often they are unable to treat the pathological features that are causative. They are often very effective, however, in treating functional cardiac disturbances such as arrhythmias, diminished contractibility, hypotension, and pain.

In summary, physicians who adopt a functional approach to the assessment and treatment of the demented patient, in conjunction with a disease-oriented approach, will be able to maintain the patient and the patient's needs as paramount; they will thereby be able to avoid the neglect that often befalls patients unfortunate enough to suffer from untreatable diseases that cause dementia. A thorough functional assessment in these patients will uncover virtually none in whom there are no opportunities for therapeutic intervention and virtually none in whom some benefit will not accrue from the physician's efforts. Without question, cognitive losses may be unyielding, and improvement in other functions may be unspectacular. Without question, family members and other caretakers may appear, in some instances, to benefit more directly than does the patient. Adoption of such an approach will, however, open for the physician unsuspected avenues in which the art of medical practice can be called fully into play.

References

1. Hakin, S., Adams, R.D. The special clinical problem of symptomatic hydrocephalus with normal cerebrospinal fluid pressure: observations on cerebrospinal fluid hydrodynamics. *J. Neurol. Sci.* 2:307-327, 1965.

2. Adams, R.D., Fisher, C.M., Hakin, S., et al. Symptomatic occult hydrocephalus with "normal" cere-

brospinal-fluid pressure: as treatable syndrome. *N. Engl. J. Med.* 273:117-126, 1965.

3. Marsden, C.D., Harrison, M.J.G. Outcome of investigation of patients with presenile dementia. *Br. Med. J.* 2:249-252, 1972.

4. Wells, C.E. Diagnosis of dementia. *Psychosomatics* 20:517-522, 1979.

5. Nott, P.N., Fleminger, J.J. Presenile dementia: the difficulties of early diagnosis. *Acta Psychiatr. Scand.* 51:210-217, 1975.

6. Ron, M.A., Toone, B.K., Garralda, M.E., et al. Diagnostic accuracy in presenile dementia. *Br. J. Psychiatry* 134:161-168, 1979.

7. Kiloh, L.G. Pseudo-dementia. *Acta Psychiatr. Scand.* 37:336-351, 1961.

8. Wells, C.E. Pseudodementia. *Am. J. Psychiatry* 136:895-900, 1979.

9. Tomlinson, B.E., Blessed, G., Roth, M. Observations on the brains of demented old people. *J. Neurol. Sci.* 11:205-242, 1970.

10. Seltzer, B., Sherwin, I. "Organic brain syndromes": an empirical study and critical review. *Am. J. Psychiatry* 135:13-21, 1979.

THE MENTALLY RETARDED: A NEED FOR UNDERSTANDING

Howard Cohen and Jane Cohen

"Concern for the parents' and siblings' well-being, receptiveness to ongoing questions, and understanding the need for further education concerning the nature of the disease process all serve to identify the caretaker who does, in fact, care."[1]

Eric was a beautiful baby and seemed to us perfect in every way. When our fourth child was born, we considered ourselves confident, almost casual, parents, having watched his three older siblings progress normally through the stages of babyhood. Although Eric's development was slower than the others—he did not walk alone until nineteen months—we were not overly concerned. However, a somewhat glazed "look" and absent speech patterns at twenty-one months caused us to suspect that there might be something vaguely wrong. We turned to our pediatrician for advice.

We had chosen for our children's doctor a man who had been practicing more than forty years and was also a family friend; he and Eric's grandfather, a physician himself, had maintained close ties for decades. This pediatrician had obviously seen a wide range of problems throughout the years of his busy practice, and he pointed out to us how much the science of pediatrics had progressed since he graduated from medical school. Not unexpectedly, he scoffed at the suggestion that Eric's development might be abnormal and was quick to reassure us that we had no cause for alarm. Looking back on that meeting, we wish there had been some doubt or equivocation on his part, for denial by Eric's primary medical caretaker made the eventual diagnosis of mental retardation all the more devastating for us, his parents. Concern on his part, at that point, for *our* concern would have enabled us to prepare gradually for the grief process through which he knew even then we would have to pass. As an aside, we discovered years later that this pediatrician himself had had a Down's syndrome son confined in an institution from birth—a well-kept secret which helps to explain his attitude toward mental retardation. Since that revelation, we have considered ourselves lucky that this doctor did not make an earlier mental retardation diagnosis and suggest institutionalization for Eric!

Our first pediatrician retired shortly after the incident related, and we transferred the care of the children to his younger associate. We reiterated our questions regarding Eric's progress and again were reassured. But our doubts persisted, and an interview was requested with a pediatric neurologist. By this time, Eric was twenty-seven months old, and it seemed to us that his obviously delayed development in many areas would lend itself to a specific diagnosis by such a specialist.

Unfortunately, our own dearth of medical sophistication and knowledge of mental retardation precluded our discovering any meaningful information from this physician. We left his office more bewildered than we had entered it. Twelve years later, when Eric, at his school's request, was reevaluated by the same neurologist, he gave us the diagnosis of "your average everyday garden-variety retardate." We then realized that our initial confusion was due in large measure to his crass insensitivity.

Several months after the initial neurologic interview, an appointment for a complete evaluation was made with the director of a hospital serving mentally and physically handicapped children. The diagnosis made that day had an aura of such finality about it that it left us completely bereft of all hope. Even if parents are prepared for the emotion-laden words "mentally retarded," surely a physician whose practice involves labeling handicapped children has an obligation to have philosophical and pragmatic information at the ready to help provide "safe passage" to the patient and his stricken family. Instead, we received a detailed litany of Eric's projected limitations (as a child and adult) and the admonition to take him home to learn to live with it. "Write him off; he's helpless" seemed to be the clear message. The lack of compassion and distance on the part of this doctor were devastating to us. A mother and physician has aptly described a more reasonable approach: "While you don't throw wet rags, you can't toss out false balloons of hope either. It's your child, and you have every right to know the facts. We have no right to keep them from you. But the doctor has to let the parent know the positives, too."[2]

Here was a problem that we would have to live with all our lives and which would even survive us, but we had been given no hint of how to cope with it or even where to turn for help. Only the severity of the prognosis was made unmistakably clear.

Perhaps we, as Eric's parents, appeared to the external world as "in control" even in the face of such overwhelming news and, therefore, not in need of support. For the conspiracy of silence extended beyond the physician and medical community—even to family and friends. One of our sisters could never bring herself to offer any consolation to us and to this day does not utter the dread words "mentally retarded." Many of our close friends will not or cannot ask after Eric's progress, as they do for our other children, and one or two even ignore his presence in the same room. Must one scream in a primal way to bring a response?

Happily, there are many more support services set up to help the mentally retarded today than there were twelve years ago. Then our pediatrician knew little about what the community had to offer, and we had great difficulty in discovering suitable programs for Eric. Like all parents of handicapped children, we have had to deal with a myriad of self-labeled professionals, with some of whom we were very impressed; others disappointed us with lack of or mis-information, failure to follow up on promises of many kinds, and patronizing attitudes. We discovered early that parents need an advocate to help them manage the needs of their retarded child—needs which change constantly, necessitating new choices by the parents. They should have an expert who knows the child well and is familiar with the resources of the community to provide the requisite diagnostic, treatment, education, and other support services for the particular problem. Ideally, that expert should be the child's pediatrician. Ours, although a specialist in learning and development problems, and chosen by us for that very reason, has never fulfilled the role or been able to refer us to someone who could. Any course of action taken in Eric's behalf has been as the result of diligent research by his parents, which, although enthusiastically undertaken, may not always have been the right step at that particular stage of his development.

For example, through a newspaper article, we learned that a psychologist at a leading hospital seemed to be having some success using behavior modification techniques with very young mentally retarded children. It was an experimental program requiring that Eric live at the hospital for five days a week for a year. Our pediatrician, although on staff, knew little about this activity but had no specific objection to Eric's participation. Although the program and its creator were controversial and generated some hostility from other departments in the hospital, we decided to try it. There was much manipulation of data and graphs, more to the enhancement of programmatic results than to the enrichment of the children involved. The psychologist, moreover, pursued successfully a better position at another institution, treating the children as if they were test-tube substances to be discarded when the data became superfluous. We emerged from this experience with the perception, reconfirmed through the years, that many professionals are more interested in using their research to enhance their careers and impress their peers, than in helping the clients who contribute to their projects and so desperately need their help.

Eric, now almost sixteen, leads a relatively normal existence, living at home with his two brothers and two sisters, and going to his special school by bus each day. He also attends a day camp in the summer designed for retarded youngsters and eagerly looks forward to all of his planned activities. We have tried to develop strong emotional ties between him and his siblings, and although he can be annoying to them (and us, too), his brothers and sisters consistently have shown their genuine love and concern for him. Years ago, a therapist gave us some simple and excellent advice: never make the other children feel neglected or deprived because of Eric, so they will not resent him. We have tried diligently to follow this sound guidance. We feel our children have been enriched by Eric's presence, sharing an experience that few have. And being an intimate part of the family, living in a loving, caring home, has meant much to Eric's own development as a person. No incarcerating institution could ever provide the positive reinforcement of such a household as Eric's, and we are convinced that this is the reason his behavior is so superior to his intelligence quotient. His closeness to his siblings also bodes well for Eric's future, when his parents will no longer be able to look after his welfare.

Being mentally retarded is only one of Eric's qualities. He has others that are more positive, such as being always cheerful, responsive, affectionate, outgoing, and vitally interested in everything going on about him. He is a constant reminder that the worth and beauty of a person lies in their presence and not in their ultimate skills.

References

1. Butler, A.B. Compassionate pediatrics. There's

something wrong with Michael: a pediatrician-mother's perspective. *Pediatrics* 71:44, 1983.

2. Jablow, M.M. *Cara*. Philadelphia: Temple University Press, 1983, p. 9.

COUNSELING AND SUPPORT FOR FAMILIES WITH GENETIC DISEASES

Ann P. Garber and David L. Rimoin

Genetic disorders can involve all body systems through a wide variety of pathogenic mechanisms. They pose a number of distinct problems for the patient and their families that must be addressed in a humanistic manner with empathy and understanding. The unique features of genetic diseases will be addressed in this essay.

Patients will usually approach the health provider with concerns about the presence of, or risk for, a genetic disease in themselves or in a present or future child. In addition to providing a diagnosis, medical prognosis, and therapy the patient should be given a clear understanding of the etiology of the disorder, the risk of recurrence in future and present family members, and approaches to its prevention. Genetic counseling, however, does not end with patient education. Counselors must also provide care for the patient's emotional needs regarding heritable disorders. Patients seeking genetic counseling are frequently in states of shock, anxiety, anger, guilt, and mourning; the physician must be prepared to deal with such emotional turmoil effectively.

Guilt and low self-esteem are common underlying feelings in many genetic counseling patients. Parents with an affected child often perceive themselves as genetically flawed individuals, responsible for creating a tragic life for their child. The idea of being defective often leads parents to feel inadequate and undesirable as mates. Feelings of guilt and low self-esteem may be even more profound once the parents have knowledge as to the mode of transmission of that inherited condition. Such feelings can be ameliorated if the counselor openly and tactfully discusses guilt with the parents and provides an honest and supportive atmosphere, while explaining mechanisms of inheritance. In some instances, this task is relatively simple, as the patient's preconceived ideas about the risk of recurrence may be far greater than his actual risk. For example, the patient may feel that the risk of the recurrence of a disorder in his offspring is very high, whereas in actuality it may be negligible. In such instances, provision of the facts may be sufficient to relieve the anxiety and guilt. In other instances, however, the perceived risk for recurrence may be realistic or even underestimated. These risk figures must be discussed with the patient at their own level of education and understanding and frequently repeated, so that the counseler is confident that the true risk is understood. It is also helpful to summarize these risks in writing so that the patients can review them periodically.

Feelings of guilt and anger often surface during such counseling sessions. This is especially true when the disorder can be traced to one parent, such as in the following situations: a) in X-linked disorders, where the mother is a carrier, b) in autosomal dominant disorders, especially where the affected parent may have a mild form of the disorder and was unaware that they were affected, or c) in chromosomal translocation syndromes, where one partner is a clinically normal balanced translocation carrier. In autosomal recessive disorders, where both parents are carriers, questions about the choice of their mate may arise, threatening the stability of the marriage, when the parents learn that they would have likely escaped having an affected child had they chosen another partner. The clinician must be prepared to deal with these feelings and aid the family in working through them.

Another unique aspect of genetic counseling is the need for the clinician to assess and provide risk information to other family members. In some cases, contact with relatives may be difficult due to estranged family relations. Frequently, the burden of the disorder leads some relatives to break family ties or avoid the truth because they are embarrassed by, or wish to deny the existence of, genetic disease in the family. Detailed explanation of the probability of recurrence in other family members is extremely important to prevent expression of the disease in the offspring of unknown carriers of the condition. The patient or parents must be educated as to their responsibility in directing this information to their at-risk relatives and provide the contact between the relative and the counselor.

Genetic diseases may first present themselves in the adult, child, newborn, or fetus. Each of these circumstances presents unique problems which will be addressed individually. A few selected problems will be described.

The Affected Adult

The clinician must be aware of the impact on the adult who is found to have a genetic disorder. In addition to offering a diagnosis, prognosis, and recurrence risk, the clinician must be prepared to deal with the emotional effect of this information on the patient. The patient frequently reacts with shock, anger, and anxiety to the knowledge that he has a progressive disease and "bad genes." His immediate reaction may well differ if he is the first in the family with the condition and thus has no personal experience with this disorder, as opposed to the situation where he is already familiar with the disease because of an affected parent or other relative. However, in both situations, in addition to the provision of risk figures and methods of prevention, the clinician must explain the prognosis and variability of the condition as well as its therapy, so that the patient will have a realistic appreciation of his future. Referral to self-help groups like the Neurofibromatosis Foundation may be useful in helping the patient gain the necessary experience with the condition, as well as providing invaluable support from other affected individuals. If the person has other affected relatives, the variability of the disorder must be addressed, as his experience with the condition may be quite biased due to an exceptionally mildly or severely affected relative. Anger and aggressive feelings toward the parent who passed on the condition may lead the patient to express hostility during the genetic counseling session. If angry feelings are not expressed, it is worthwhile to tactfully elicit such feelings rather than let the patient conceal the anger and consequently suffer the suppressed and unresolved hostility.

Regardless of the patient's previous experience with

his condition, his self-image will likely be affected by the presentation of a genetic diagnosis. Body image is frequently distorted and overemphasizes deformity. Understandably, neurofibromatosis patients with a mild to moderate lesion are horrified to be categorized with "The Elephant Man" and as a result may develop a distorted body concept. If not dealt with, poor body image can negatively affect the patient's emotions, pride, overall confidence, and ability to function. It is important to encourage physically deformed patients to discuss their feelings about their handicap and help them to minimize the effect on their outlook on life. It must be stressed that genetic counseling involves painful issues and requires the physician to give the patient time and consideration.

A particularly controversial issue is that of pre-clinical detection of late-onset dominant conditions, such as Huntington's disease. In most affected families, onset is in the 30s or 40s, and an at-risk individual would have to be symptomless beyond age 60 to conclude that he would have little chance of being affected. Because of the severe and tragic prognosis of Huntington's disease, and because at-risk individuals are often not aware of their future disease status at the time of marriage and family planning, pre-clinical detection of the condition has been attempted. The physician faces a dilemma: should he allow an affected individual 20 years of blissful ignorance, or should he tell the symptomless patient that he is definitely affected? If pre-clinical testing is not done, 50% of at-risk, but unaffected individuals, will live in needless fear of developing this disorder, and those who are affected may have several children before realizing that they have Huntington's disease. Pre-clinical testing, however, may be inadequate or inaccurate in picking out all carriers of the gene of Huntington's disease or other late-onset disorders, further compounding the controversy surrounding this topic.

In addition to discussing feelings about the patient's disease and diagnosis, the question of reproduction must be addressed. If this is a dominant disorder with a 50% risk of recurrence, the patient's decision as to whether to reproduce or avoid reproduction is greatly influenced by his own self-image and ability to cope with the disorder. In this instance, issues of birth control and/or prenatal diagnosis and abortion are quite different than with the unaffected parents of a child with a recessive disease, as the individual with a dominant disorder is, in essence, deciding whether or not to "clone" himself or, in the case of abortion, whether to "kill" his clone. If he chooses to avoid reproduction, what are his feelings about himself, in terms of self-worth, desire to be alive, etc.? Each of these issues must be addressed, and these feelings should be provoked and allowed to air themselves prior to reproductive decision-making. If the couple desires to have children, but are unwilling to take the chance of having an affected offspring or to abort an affected fetus if prenatal diagnosis is available, artificial insemination or the future possibilities of ovum transfer should be discussed. Obviously, these alternate methods of reproduction will elicit a new set of emotional responses, but in selected couples, they may prove to be their best option.

The Affected Child

When the patient found to have a newly diagnosed genetic disease is a child who was previously normal as a newborn and infant, the family is faced with a variety of emotional issues. In addition to the shock of learning that their beloved child has a chronic, debilitating, or perhaps lethal disorder, when the genetic nature of the disorder is defined, the parents will often feel guilty and responsible for causing the disease in their child, and then develop low self-esteem by considering themselves genetically flawed and perhaps inadequate as mates and parents. Such feelings must be identified and explored with the couple as they work through their shock, anxiety, anger, denial, and final acceptance of the situation. The immediate situation will obviously differ if this is the first affected child in the family or if previous children or their relatives were affected. In all instances, a clear understanding of the prognosis and variability of the disorder must be provided, in addition to plans of management and therapy. Genetic counseling concerning risks and potential methods of prevention, such as prenatal diagnosis, may offer new hope to the distressed parents and should be addressed as early as possible. In addition to their concern with bearing future affected offspring, they will also have fears of the disease appearing in their other apparently well children, as well as in their future grandchildren. In many instances, these fears will be unfounded genetically or can be discounted following careful examination and/or pre-clinical testing of their other children. These studies and subsequent genetic counseling should be provided as soon as possible in order to limit their concerns to the affected child in question.

In the case of the older child, one must deal with his feelings of being affected with a chronic, debilitating, or deforming disease. In most instances, they will be no different than the conerns of a child with a nongenetic disorder, unless he has had previous experience with the disease in an older sibling or relative. In such instances, one must be aware of his identification with the older affected relative, discuss the variability of the disorder, and hopefully, the possibility that he may not end up as severely affected. Utilizaton of self-help groups such as the Little People of America can be of great value in helping the child accept his condition, learn that he is not alone in the world, and develop adult models for success in life. In the older child or teenager, discussion of risk of recurrence in his future children must also be undertaken.

The Affected Newborn

Frequently, the afflicted newborn is the first family member known to have genetic disease. When parents are confronted with the emotional crisis which accompanies malformation or retardation in the newborn, experienced counselors should be called on to provide help. The immediate needs of parents can be broken down into three broad categories: 1) to understand the etiology of the disorder, 2) to understand the recurrence risk of the disorder, and 3) to obtain psychological and emotional support needed to help cope with the birth of an affected baby.

Effective communication of the diagnosis to new parents is dependent on the quality of the physician's presentation, the intelligence of the parents, and the psychosocial state of the parents. The parents' anxiety caused by their realization that their baby "has something wrong" is understandably heightened when the physician devotes special attention to providing them with "the facts." Counseling at this time should be simple, supportive, and straightforward. Parents in such acute grief and shock are not able to concentrate on complex explanations, but will often be reassured knowing that information is available and will be thoroughly discussed with them at a more appropriate time.

The immediate reactions experienced by parents of an affected child are shock, disbelief, denial, and rejection. However, even after parents have begun to accept the situation, longer-term reactions are often present. The most common emotion brought on by an affected child is sorrow, but it does not appear that sorrow can be signficantly assuaged through counseling. The physician who counsels parents with long-term sorrow should be aware that this is a natural reaction and encourage the parents to accept it as such. However, if acute grief appears excessive or persists beyond several months, psychiatric consultation should be obtained.

Guilt feelings are particularly strong when responsibility can be assigned to one parent or the other. Self-reproach, shame, and a diminished self-esteem frequently ensue. Physicians should elicit guilt feelings from patients and help assuage the guilt by providing an honest, yet supportive, and non-threatening atmosphere for discussion of such feelings. Anger experienced by one or both parents is often directed to the marital partner, the child, toward God, or toward one's self. Counseling is an important process for parents with acute anger; clinicians should help parents acknowledge their anger and, hopefully, allow them to let go of it and seek support from family and close friends.

In those genetic disorders presenting in the newborn with significant mental retardation or multiple severe malformations, the question arises as to the immediate care of the child and whether he should be taken home, institutionalized, or given up for foster care. Although in the majority of instances the child will be taken home from the nursery when stabilized, in certain cases institutionalization should be considered. The family should be made aware of all options available to them. The physician must carefully examine the parents' own family situation and ability to cope with the burden of the severely retarded or malformed child. It is frequently helpful if the physician himself brings this matter up initially, stating that there is no right or wrong answer to placement and the correct decision depends upon the particular family's circumstances. Although it may superficially appear best to have the parents take the child home and directly experience their ability to cope with the situation, guilt about placement may increase as bonding with the child occurs. An immediate decision for placement is more common when the child has significant bodily or facial deformities, as opposed to those instances where the newborn appears physically normal or only mildly deformed, but severe mental retardation is a certainty. It is important to offer the parents an accurate and objective description of the prognosis and avoid giving them false hopes for the future. Utilization of pictures of similarly affected individuals or even introduction to parents of other affected children may be helpful. Whatever their decision, physician support is extremely important during this difficult time and in the years ahead.

In addition to the question concerning placement of the severely retarded newborn, the clinician is also frequently confronted with the difficult issue of whether to provide or withhold "heroic" therapy. This issue has recently received a great deal of attention in the American media with the so-called "Baby Doe" regulations. The physician will likely have strong personal views on this subject, which might be quite different from those of the parents. Whose beliefs are to be followed in such situations? If the parents, after fully understanding the prognosis, desire that all medical therapy possible be provided for the child, there is little question that all routine therapy should be provided. If, however, the parents do not wish to subject their retarded infant to "life-saving" surgery and wish to let "nature take its course," should their wishes be respected, even if one or more members of the medical or nursing team feel differently? Unfortunately, there is no clear ethical answer to this dilemma. It appears that stringent legal regulations may necessitate such therapy in all instances in the future. If this cookbook method of dealing with such an emotionally charged area becomes law, the clinician will have to help the parents deal with the issue and explore means of financing the care and perhaps the placement of the child. If we are able to take a more humanistic approach to each individual case and fully explore the parents' feelings and respect their informed decision, the clinician may well have to serve as the parents' advocate, if he agrees with their position. If he does not agree with their decision, however, there is a major question as to whether he ought to withdraw from the case and allow the parents to engage someone with more compatible feelings.

Following the birth of an affected child, many parents choose to avoid having any further children or to divorce because of the fear of having another affected offspring. Discussion of the available methods of prevention of recurrence of the particular disease can offer immediate hope to many parents. With the major advances in prenatal diagnosis through amniocentesis and ultrasound, many genetic disorders can be detected *in utero*, and the affected child aborted if the parents so desire. The limitations of prenatal diagnosis, however, must also be addressed, stating that one can only detect the particular disorder one is testing for and that any pregnancy bears a 2 to 4% risk of producing a child with some birth defect.

The Affected Fetus

Although the great majority of couples utilizing prenatal diagnosis can be reassured that the fetus is not affected, when the fetus is found to be abnormal, the physician must be prepared to deal with a wide range of emotional reactions. The couple's immediate reaction to the question of selective abortion of an affected fetus is dependent on a number of factors, including their religious and moral feelings about abortion in general, their relative fertility, their desire for this pregnancy, and the experience with the disorder detected. Abortion for genetic indications represents the loss of a wanted pregnancy. It is likely that, although abortion is preferable to the birth of an affected child to many couples, few couples truly anticipate that an abortion will be necessary. If the couple has had relative infertility and has attempted to achieve a pregnancy for a long time, the decision to abort the fetus is extremely difficult. If the couple is opposed to abortion on religious grounds and finds that these feelings change when confronted with the affected fetus, it is important to explore these feelings carefully and perhaps obtain the help of the couple's clergy.

When the parents have had amniocentesis because of a previously affected child with Tay Sachs disease or Down's syndrome, for example, they have had personal experience with the burden and tragedy of the disorder and have chosen to undergo amniocentesis because of their desire to prevent having further affected children. If they have had prenatal diagnosis because of belonging to a high-risk group, but have not had previous experience with a disorder, they should have at least had pre-amniocentesis genetic counseling and be somewhat prepared for the decision at hand. One can never predict, however, the patient's actual reaction to detection of an abnormal fetus, regardless of their preparedness for the diagnosis and their previously stated attitude toward termination of pregnancy.

When a diagnosis is made in a fetus, intensive counseling must be performed and the parents made to work through their feelings with a realistic outlook on the prognosis of the child if it should be born. With the increasing sophistication of ultrasound techniques and with more routine use of ultrasound during pregnancy, a number of fetuses with structural malformations are now being detected, without any prior warning. This presents an especially acute, emotionally charged situation, since the parents must be counseled and decisions concerning abortion made relatively quickly due to the limitations of gestational age and termination. The parents, who are usually quite excited about the pregnancy and have already experienced quickening and bonding to the fetus, must be told their fetus is abnormal, be made aware of the clinical features and prognosis of the disorder with which they have probably had no experience, and given genetic counseling concerning their future risks.

In addition to all of these unique features of genetic counseling for a disease detected in a fetus, the parents will usually experience the same reactions as they would with the detection of an abnormal newborn or child including shock, anger, anxiety, denial, guilt, and loss of self-esteem. It is imperative that the couple's physician and counselors spend a great deal of time with the parents to help them through this difficult period.

In summary, families with genetic disease have a number of unique problems and emotional reactions that must be dealt with sympathetically. The physician must not only be prepared to make a diagnosis, manage the case medically, and offer genetic risk figures, but deal with the family's feelings of guilt, anger, anxiety, sorrow, and loss of self-esteem. Collaboration with a well-trained and sensitive genetic counselor may be most helpful in achieving these goals and helping the family understand and cope with the situation in the best possible manner.

References

Applebaum, E.G. and Firestein, S.K. *A Genetic Counseling Casebook*. New York: The Free Press, 1983.

Fletcher, J.C. *Coping with Genetic Disorders—A Guide for Clergy and Parents*. San Francisco: Harper and Row, 1982.

Hsia, Y.E., Hirschhorn, K., Silverberg, R.L., and Godmilow, L. (eds.). *Counseling in Genetics*. New York: Alan R. Liss, Inc., 1979.

WHAT CAN I DO FOR A DYING FRIEND?*

David Rabin and Pauline L. Rabin

At some time in our lives, we all encounter serious illness in a relative, friend, or colleague. Sympathy and support are natural responses expressed easily to the stricken person during an acute medical setback. Illness of a progressive or terminal nature extending over months or years provokes uncertainty about how we should pursue our relations with the sick person. We are all threatened to some degree by confrontation with severe disease or impending death. This forces us to face the inescapable truth that all life is finite including our own. Our emotional equilibrium can be so disturbed by another's illness that the instinctive and self-protective response is to withdraw.

---

* Dedicted to the Memory of Eugene Meyer, III, M.D., Physician, Teacher, and Humanitarian.

There is, however, a conflict between this visceral, often subconscious, response and the humane desire to show love and compassion for those who suffer. Tentative approaches are made to the patient and the family. The patient may appear uncomfortable; the spouse may become emotional. We conclude that our actions have been unhelpful, perhaps intrusive, and that we should respect the privacy of the patient and his family. However inadvertently, this reasoning is the beginning of isolation for the patient.

To this point, we have considered the reactions of those who are healthy. Let us now reflect on the spectrum of emotions experienced by the patient. The late Dr. Eugene Meyer, III, Professor of Psychiatry and Medicine at Johns Hopkins Hospital, was a pioneer in the field of liaison psychiatry. He made regular bedside rounds on the Osler Medical Service, and relating to dying patients he frequently emphasized the following two precepts. First, the universal response to loss of health is grief which is characterized by sadness, tearfulness, and irritability. Secondly, the patient may be afraid to die, but his immediate and overriding concerns are fear of enduring pain, loss of dignity, and isolation.

Knowing all this, how can we help a dying friend? For most patients loneliness and alienation are hard to endure. The patient needs a sense that people care, and you can show your interest and concern by asking to visit your friend. Never rely on signals alone, which can be totally misleading. If a visit is inconvenient or if the patient prefers seclusion, let him or his family tell you. Some patients withdraw permanently from interactions with others, and this must be respected. Meyer stressed that, under these circumstances, it is particularly important to provide support and comfort to the patient's family who must cope with the tragedy. This also applies in situations when the patient's faculties or level of consciousness are impaired. It is wise to remember that circumstances do not remain static. Pain and depression intensified by adverse changes in appearance, confinement to bed, or incoherent speech may have made the patient uncomfortable with people. With the passage of time, some patients overcome their depression and once more wish to resume social contact. You will not be aware of the change in attitude unless you remain in touch with the family. It is also up to the patient and the family to let friends know when company would be welcome.

You may feel very tense before the visit, particularly if a long interval has elapsed since your last contact. You may be unaware of the precise state of your friend's health. A small symbol of caring, such as flowers or candy, and the accompanying grace of giving and receiving, will ease those first stressful moments. As you reach out to the family in distress, their sadness and awkwardness should not be misinterpreted as a rejection. You will be apprehensive as to what to say, but your presence alone will constitute support. Try to avoid coming on strong with pressured talk or false reassurances about how well the patient appears to be. It is preferable to say, "I hope you are reasonably comfortable today." Give the patient the choice whether or not to talk about his illness. After some initial discomfort, you will usually find that your friendship is unchanged, and subjects of mutual interest continue to be compelling and enjoyable to discuss.

What can you do for a dying friend? Recognize that he is still alive and that he and his family cherish human contact and bonds of friendship.

DEATH AND DYING

Patrick B. Friel

Attitudes toward death have changed dramatically over the centuries. Death had been viewed as a natural event to be accepted without undue fear, and presided over by the dying persons. In recent times, however, death has been transformed into a lonely and frequently painful ordeal occurring in the isolation of a hospital room, presided over by the physician and other health care personnel. In the course of a terminal illness, the role of the physician should change from curing to caring. This role needs a full understanding of the various adaptive stages involved in facing death, from initial denial to ultimate acceptance. The physician must also appreciate the various components, both physical and psychological, that constitute the pain of dying.

Lord Francis Bacon,[1] the 17th-century English philosopher and Lord Chancellor, wrote, "It is as natural to die as to be born." More recently Alexander Solzhenitsyn[2] described those facing death as dying easily "as if they were just moving into a new house." Such familiar resignation contrasts sharply with the angry denial that is more typical of the contemporary scene.

WESTERN ATTITUDES TOWARD DEATH

Phillipe Aries[3] points out that in the beginning man apparently did not fear death; most commonly the person was forewarned and knew when and how he was going to die. Death was accepted without fear, as being part of the natural progression. Death was neither hastened nor delayed. Certain rituals were carried out, liturgies were created, and customs became established. Thus prepared, the dying person carried out the final steps of the traditional death ceremony as was prescribed. It is particularly noteworthy that the dying person knew and presided over the protocol involved in dying. This situation existed for a millennium. Dying was a public event and death took place in the presence of family, friends, neighbors, and children.

From the Middle Ages to the mid-19th century, the attitude toward death changed from something that was commonplace, ordinary, expected, and accepted, to something that was shameful and forbidden. Lies began to surround the process of dying. Motivation for lies surrounding death was at first a desire to spare the sick person but rapidly changed to a new sentiment more characteristic of modern times: the topic of death had to be avoided not for the sake of the dying, but for the sake of society and those close to the dying one. The strong emotion caused by what was now the ugliness of death had to be avoided. Beginning around 1930, the evolution regarding death underwent marked acceleration and an important change took place. People no longer died at home; the place of death became the hospital or the nursing home. Dying in the presence of one's family was no longer acceptable. Death took place frequently in a hospital room, and all too often alone.

At the turn of the century, two thirds of the people who died in this country were under the age of fifty; most died at home in their beds surrounded by their family and friends. Children learned to view death as a part of life, not threatening or unusual, but simply a part of reality. Today most deaths occur in an older population, those over sixty-five years of age, and two thirds of our people die in medical institutions and nursing homes. Most children are not exposed to death in their formative years when they have the security and comfort of their family to help them deal with it. That they may have difficulty coping with death when they become adults is not surprising.

Geoffrey Gorer[4] states that death became a taboo in the 20th century and replaced sex as a forbidden subject. In former times, he writes, children were told they were brought by the stork but were admitted to the farewell scene at the bed of the dying person. Today children are initiated in their early years to the physiology of love, but when friends or relatives die, they are told bizarre fantasies to explain away the death. It appears the more society became liberated from Victorian constraints on sex, the more it developed constraints centering around the subject of death (referred to as "the pornography of death" by Gorer).

HUMANISM IN MEDICINE

In recent centuries, Western civilization has been influenced and shaped by a system of thought variously called scientific, rational, or mechanistic. This system has helped in creating a technology that has brought enormous material advances to much of the world. Medicine as practiced today reflects this method of thought and relies on the technology it has produced. This technology and approach can seem cold and out of place when it comes to caring for the dying. Dr. Frederick Stenn,[5] an associate professor of medicine at Northwestern Medical School in Chicago, wrote on his death bed:

> The other day, my doctor sat at my bedside just to talk. He assured me my physical complaints will be eased and that he will be in regular attendance. We talked frankly of the dying process and the need of living as I am dying, living to fully appreciate every moment of life. I like our conversations but it is hard to come by. Most physicians have lost the pearl that was once an intimate part of medicine, and that is humanism. Machinery, efficiency and precision have driven from the heart warmth, compassion, sympathy, and concern for the individual. Medicine is now an icy science; its charm belongs to another age. The dying man can get little comfort from the mechanical doctor.

THE ACCEPTANCE PROCESS

By understanding the various stages and processes involved in the progression from life to death, we can bring compassion, sympathy, and concern to the dying person. Dr. Kübler-Ross[6] and her associates have contributed greatly to our understanding of what the dying person experiences. Kübler-Ross describes five stages in the process: denial, anger, bargaining, depression, and acceptance. As any student of medicine knows, patients do not always follow the textbook pattern, and so too with dying patients. In the course of a fairly lengthy illness, most patients progress through the various stages, but in shorter illnesses the stages may be condensed, varied, or skipped, and indeed some patients do not give up almost total denial until the end.

The Denial Stage

When a patient is told or realizes that he or she is dying, there is not total comprehension of the implications of that knowledge. Such knowledge would be too painful for the patient to bear. Death is a universal threat, and when it becomes a probability, a device is needed that prevents the intrusion of the fearful meaning of death into the patient's consciousness. Characteristically, the dying person's initial reaction is denial. Denial in this context is an adjustment reaction that has been defined as "the repudiation of part or all of the available meaning of an event for the purpose of minimizing fear and anxiety."[7] There is a time in the course of an illness when denial is encouraged and used advantageously in the relief of the patient's distress. There is another time, however, when this reaction is unacceptable and ineffective. The attitudes of the physician and others who care for the patient play a vital role in determining whether denial will be used effectively. When the reality of the situation permits legitimate optimism, hopefulness on the part of the physician and other attending personnel will help and encourage the patient in the use of denial. When optimism has no basis in fact, medical personnel have a duty to help the patient face reality rather than let him face this frightening experience alone. Meaningful optimism and hope must be founded on truth, but when truth dictates the inevitability of death, the patient must be assisted in facing the inevitable.

The first reaction to catastrophic news that threatens the universal unconscious concept of immortality is "No—it's not true, it can't be me," but this reaction has to give way to the realization, "It is me; it was not a mistake." Very few patients are able to maintain a make-believe world in which they are healthy and well until they die. When the early stages of denial cannot be maintained any longer, they are replaced by feelings of anger, rage, envy, and resentment. Patients begin to ask, "Why me?" and at this stage harbor fantasies of why it should be someone else, someone seemingly less worthy of life than themselves.

The Anger Stage

In contrast to the stage of denial, the stage of anger is difficult for family and staff to cope with, because the patient's anger is displaced and projected at times almost at random. The attending physician is criticized for being incompetent or not prescribing the right medications. Nurses are also the target of anger. Whatever they touch is not right. The moment they leave the room the bell rings, but when they return to adjust the pillow or straighten out the bed, they are blamed for never leaving the patient alone. Family visits are received with little cheerfulness and anticipation, and often lead to painful encounters. In an effort to avoid further pain and grief, the family generally cuts the visits short or comes less frequently, reactions that only increase the patient's discomfort and anger.

The problem is that few people place themselves in the patient's position and wonder where anger comes from. Most people would be angry if their life's activities, their hopes, dreams, goals, and aspirations were going to be interrupted. It is only natural that the anger is going to be vented on people likely to enjoy all the things that the dying person will soon be denied. The patient who is respected and understood, difficult as this may be, and is given attention and time, will soon lower his voice and reduce his angry demands. The patient will come to realize that he is still treated as a valuable human being, cared for, and allowed to function at the highest possible level as long as he can. The patient will realize that he will be listened to without the need for a temper tantrum and will be visited without having to ring the bell. The tragedy in many situations like this is that the reasons for the patient's anger are not understood but are taken personally, when in fact the anger has little or nothing to do with the people who are its target. If the staff or the patient's family react personally to the anger, they are only increasing the patient's difficulty and feeding the hostile behavior. If the family does not understand, they may react by using avoidance, shortening their visits, or getting into unnecessary arguments by defending their actions when in fact these matters are not directly related to the source of the patient's anger.

The Bargaining Stage

As the patient comes to realize that anger has not changed the unacceptable reality, there is a tendency to revert to a device frequently used by children, to bargain. Children in this way often hope to wrest from their parents a special privilege that has been denied. The dying patient hopes it possible to negotiate a quid-pro-quo solution. There is often a promise to abandon venality or undertake heroic service to placate God or benefit mankind. In return, the patient hopes to obtain either a cure or a temporary prolongation of life, to permit attending a special graduation or observing a cherished anniversary. In the bargaining phase, there is an implicit promise that the patient will not ask for more if this one favor is granted. However, patients do not keep their promises. They are very much like children who promise never to be bad again. Needless to say, children will be bad and the dying person will try to arrange one more bargain.

The Depressive Stage

When the terminally ill patient has had a recurrence of serious symptoms needing rehospitalization and perhaps further surgery, and can no longer effectively deny the seriousness of the illness, depressive symptoms usually develop. Depression in the beginning often relates to the painful and disfigurative nature of radical surgery. Extensive treatment and hospitalization impose financial burdens. At first luxuries and later necessities may have to be curtailed. The cost of treatment and hospitalization may force patients to sell the only possessions they have. Patients and their families may be unable to keep a house they built for their old age or continue to send a child through college. There may be the added loss of a job due to absences entailed by illness. Mothers may have to become breadwinners, thus depriving children of the attention they previously had.

All these reasons for depression are well known to everyone who deals with terminally ill patients. This type of depression might be referred to as a reaction to the threat and the consequences of an illness. As time goes on another type of depression develops that is not related to past loss but is more an anticipation of what is to come. This depression results from the grief the terminally ill patient will feel when preparing for the final separation from the world. The patient is in the process of losing everything and everyone he loves, and it is only natural that such a threat should evoke sadness.

The treatment of these two depressions is different. The first type of depression is treated by appropriate encouragement, by trying to get the patient to look at the brighter side of life, and offering what reasonable hope can be given. However, when the depression is a tool to prepare for the impending loss of one's loved ones or to facilitate a stage of ultimate acceptance, encouragement and reassurance are no longer meaningful. In fact, the patient should not be encouraged to look at the sunny side of things for this would distract him from contemplating his impending death. It would be contradictory to tell the patient not to be sad because being sad, lonely, and depressed in the face of this impending loss is appropriate. If the patient is allowed to express sorrow, then the stage of final acceptance will be easier. This stage of depression, which is more apathy than depression, is usually silent in contrast to the earlier depression, during which the patient has much to share and needs verbal reassurance. In the second stage, there is little or no need for words. Reassurance is often more effectively expressed with a touch of the hand, a stroking of the hair, or a silent sitting together, rather than with words. This is a time when the patient begins to occupy himself with things ahead rather than with what is behind. Too much interference from visitors who try to cheer the patient hinders the necessary emotional preparation rather than enhancing it.

When the patient is preparing to die, it is unfortunate if the preparation conflicts with the physician's desires and wishes; the patient is forced to struggle for life while preparing to die. Members of the health professions should be aware of this particular stage, and help the patient deal with the discrepancies and conflicts that can exist between the patient and his environment, including his family. Physicians should know that this type of depression is necessary and beneficial if the patient is to die in a state of ultimate acceptance and peace. Patients who have been able to work through their anguish and their anxiety are able ultimately to achieve a stage of passive resignation. If this reassurance could be shared with the families, they too could be spared unnecessary anguish.

The Stage of Acceptance or Resignation

If the patient has had enough time and help in working through these various stages, he will usually reach a point where he is neither depressed nor angry about his fate. The patient will have been able to express feelings of envy for the living and the healthy, and anger at those who do not have to face their end so soon. The patient will have mourned the impending loss of so many meaningful people and places, and will contemplate the coming end with a certain degree of quiet expectation. The patient will be tired and in most cases weak, and will have a need to doze off frequently for brief periods of sleep.

Acceptance should not be mistaken for a happy stage but one almost void of feelings. It is as if the pain is gone, the struggle is over, and there is a time for rest before the final journey. At this time the family usually needs more help than the patient. The patient wishes to be left alone, his circle of interest diminishes, and he does not wish to be stirred up by news and problems of the outside world. The patient often requests that visitors be limited and that the length of visits be shortened. The television is turned off, and communication is more nonverbal than verbal. The patient may with a gesture of the hand invite those who attend him to sit down for a silent visit. Moments of silence may be the most meaningful communication for people who are comfortable in the presence of the dying person. Such visits give reassurance to the dying patient that he will not be abandoned or left alone, that it is all right to say nothing, that the important things have been taken care of and that it is only a question of time. It will reassure the patient not to be left alone when he is no longer talking; the squeeze of a hand, a look, or a nod may express that reassurance more effectively than words.

The patient's family go through stages similar to those described for the patient. That the family also needs much help and support during this process cannot be stressed too strongly. Accepting the loss of a loved one is difficult in normal circumstances, but in families racked with dissension and ambivalence this loss will be more difficult to face. Complex feelings surface and have to be dealt with; otherwise managing the dying person will be more difficult and more troublesome for those charged with this responsibility.

CHANGING EMPHASIS FROM
CURING TO CARING

A time comes in the course of chronic illness when the goal of the physician must change from curing to caring. The emphasis shifts from the disease to the patient, and from the pathology to the dying person who needs help to face death. This shift of emphasis is perhaps one of the most demanding experiences in the course of the physician's career.

Some physicians may challenge the concept that caring for a terminally ill patient needs a definite preparation for death. Physicians who view their responsibility as the prevention of death rather than the preservation of health and the relief of suffering, will look upon such a measure as defeatism. Physicians who for personal and neurotic reasons need to deny their own mortality will get caught in the counterphobic battle against death, always insisting on one more therapeutic effort. Such measures do not serve to prolong life but prolong the act of dying. The goal should be to refrain from trying to prolong life beyond its right time, and not to deliberately hasten its termination.

Determining the right time to prolong life is not always a simple clinical exercise, but can be as complex and controversial as the problem of determining the time of death. Extraneous complexities, such as the conflicting wishes of the patient's family or other members of the treatment team, can add to the difficulty. The physician should remember his primary responsibility is to the patient and that life should have the benefit of the doubt. Lamerton[8] offers some further guidelines in making this determination; he points out that patients show definite changes in their outlook and understanding, reflecting an expectation not for a cure but an assurance of care and relief from suffering. These changes surface as a better-established sense of trust, relaxation, sense of contentment, and a willingness to give up. Lamerton views this change of mind as a preparation for death.

On the other hand, the unpredictable can happen, and the clinician must be alert for rare instances when there is an unexplained arrest or regression of even a widely disseminated malignancy. The physician who can accept mortality and view death as the logical conclusion of life will best be able to discharge his duty to his patients as defined in the adage "to cure sometimes, to relieve often, but to comfort always."

MANAGEMENT OF TERMINAL PAIN

In her pioneering work on pain and its management in the terminally ill, Saunders[9] has pointed out pain's many components including the physical, mental, interpersonal, financial, and the spiritual. Unless attention is paid to all these factors, complete alleviation of pain will not be achieved. The physician who is satisfied with relieving physical pain by the use of drugs will not do justice to his or her patients. Easing pain by reducing the patient to a comatose state is not only bad medicine but is entirely unnecessary, and some might say verges on malpractice.

Physical Pain

When pain reaches the point where it disturbs the patient, relief is needed. Mild drugs and minor analgesics can be continued for as long as they are effective. As the pain becomes more constant and intense, the need for more potent analgesics can ultimately lead to the use of opiates, either in their naturally occurring or synthetic forms. The typical pain of a patient with cancer is constant and needs continual control and the routine use of drugs. The drug that seems best suited to the patient is given regularly at an effective dose level. The dose is titrated to the level of the pain of the patient so that relief is complete for the interval between doses. The patient should not be allowed to have pain or need to continually ask for relief. The dose of analgesics needs to be constantly reviewed to prevent the patient from having pain between doses. Usually drugs can be given orally; the parenteral route is needed only if the patient has chronic nausea or is unable to swallow during the last few days or even hours. The dose needed may increase but does not escalate inexorably or lead to addiction. Tolerance to the point of making the drugs ineffective does not develop. There is neither a standard nor a maximum dose of analgesia but only each patient's optimum dose, which allows him to remain both free of pain and alert until the disease itself clouds his consciousness.

Terminal pain includes forms of physical distress not generally described by the patient or physician as pain. Dyspnea, for example, can create an intolerable sensation of suffocation that can be adequately relieved with narcotics when their use is no longer contra-indicated. By using narcotics in combination with one of the phenothiazines or with benzodiazepines, this symptom can be completely abolished. For most patients with bronchopneumonia treatment with antibiotics and oxygen would be appropriate; in the aged and the dying it is often better to relieve the dyspnea with analgesics. Hygiene of the mouth is of the greatest importance to the dying patient as is the relief of constipation, which is often severe because of the constant use of opiates. There is always a place for the symptomatic relief of pain should this be drainage of an abscess, relief of acute bowel obstruction, or various neurosurgical procedures such as temporary or permanent nerve block. The emphasis should always be on relief that is appropriate to the circumstances.

Mental Anguish

Mental pain in terminal disease is a reality too often disregarded or ignored. Most typically mental anguish is a combination of anxiety and depression. Anxiety is understandable in patients who see no end to their illness and suffering. Anxiety in these circumstances usually responds more effectively to a concerned listener than it does to tranquilizers. A patient's fears are not always overtly or exclusively concerned with his illness, but whatever form the fears take they tend to lose much of their force and pain once they have been expressed in words, however incoherently. Depression and distress in the dying often stem from the fear of loneliness and the dread of isolation. Antidepressants have limited value and should be used in low dosages because of their tendency to cause confusion in the weak and the gravely ill. Again it should be emphasized that a sympathetic listener is likely to help more than most drugs; given support and encouragement patients have far greater reserves of courage and resolve than many might suspect.

Social Aspects of Pain

The gradual relinquishing of responsibilities may be one of the greatest pains that confronts a dying patient.

Who will assume responsibility for children not yet independent, or for a partner who needs life-long support? In such situations both the patient and his family are mutually bereaved, and it is difficult, perhaps even unrealistic, to separate them. The attending physician has to listen carefully to the messages and the pleas that come from both the patient and the family at this time. Difficult questions and problems surface; solutions are not easy but if possibilities are explored in an atmosphere of understanding, kindness, and honesty, then coping mechanisms will usually emerge to bring relief and comfort to the patient and the family. Much painful mutual effort is often needed to help a family move from denial to a direct confrontation with a fatal illness. One can only begin to approach these formidable problems when confidence has been gained and exchanged in the context of an ongoing relationship that includes the family. In an atmosphere of frankness there can be the sharing that brings relief from the misery of the social aspects of chronic terminal pain and death. Financial worries, including the costs of treatment for a lengthy terminal illness and the cost of supporting and maintaining those dependent on the dying person, can contribute significantly to the social aspect of pain.

The Spiritual Component

Fundamental questions regarding the meaning of life and death often surface and are dealt with in the context of the values and beliefs of the dying person. Religion and faith, supernatural or natural, play a significant and helpful role. Those attending the dying patient should never think of imposing their own religious faith on another person, especially in a time of total helplessness and dependence. However, those who attend the dying cannot help but be impressed by the sense of relief and peace that dying patients find in their different ways.

Saunders[9] writes that the needs of dying patients were summed up for all time in the seemingly simple words "Watch with me." The simplicity is perhaps misleading. The comment does not mean "take away" and it could not have meant "understand," but its most straightforward and unequivocal instruction is "Be there." The physician who is there effectively as a person and as a professional will relieve the concern of the dying expressed so well by Montaigne: "It grieves them not to be dead but to die."

References

1. Bacon, F. Of death. *Essaies of Sir Francis Bacon.* London: John Beale, 1612.

2. Solzhenitsyn, A. *The Cancer Ward.* New York: Dial Press, 1969, pp. 96-7.

3. Aries, P. *Western Attitudes Toward Death.* Baltimore and London: The Johns Hopkins University Press, 1974, pp. 1-25.

4 Gorer, G. *Death, Grief and Mourning.* New York: Anchor Books, Doubleday & Co., 1967, pp. 192-9.

5. Stenn, F. Thoughts of a dying physician. *Forum on Medicine.* 1980; 3: 718-9.

6. Kübler-Ross, E. *On Death and Dying.* New York: Macmillan Publishing Co., 1973, pp. 34-121.

7. Hackett, R.P., Weisman, A.D. Reaction to the imminence of death. In Drosser, G.H., Wechsler, H., Greenblatt, M., eds. *The Threat of Impending Disaster*. Cambridge, Mass.: MIT Press, 1964, p. 300.

8. Lamerton, R. *Care of the Dying*. Hertfordshire, England: The Garden City Press Limited, 1977, pp. 75-6.

9. Saunders, C.M. The challenge of terminal care. In Symington, T., Carter, R.L., eds. *Scientific Foundations of Oncology*. London: William Heineman Medical Books, 1975, pp. 673-8.

ACUTE GRIEF

Pauline L. Rabin and J. Kirby Pate

ABSTRACT

The purpose of this paper is to describe guidelines for physicians confronted with breaking the news to families that a loved one has unexpectedly or suddenly died in the emergency room. Doing so is difficult, but the knowledge that one is behaving professionally and humanely will help to alleviate the anxiety engendered.

THE GRIEF REACTION

Grief is a state of intense emotional suffering caused by a significant loss, disaster, or misfortune. The reactions to grief are both physiologic and psychologic

185

and are characterized by alterations in thinking, feeling, and behavior. It is conceptually helpful to divide the grief reaction into three phases. The *immediate phase* is the first reaction, extending over minutes to hours.[1] *Acute grief* develops within a few hours to days and is characterized by somatic symptoms and intense subjective distress.[2] This stage may last several weeks or months and may be delayed, exaggerated, or pathologically absent. *Mourning* is the lengthy process which begins with acute grief and extends into a period of reorganization of psychologic life, with attachment to new people and interests.[3]

We will confine our discussion to understanding the immediate phase and its management.

IMMEDIATE PHASE: PATTERNS OF REACTIONS

The impact of the news of death of a loved one leaves the family in a state of shock, and they may even try to deny the facts. A sense of numbness may be experienced as well as some temporary confusion—a dazed feeling. After a few minutes the family will become attentive and even hyperalert as they try to absorb the meaning of the news.

Clinically the immediate phase of grief is characterized by three recognizable patterns of alarm, anxiety, and anger.[4]

Alarm is the characteristic initial response to a sudden significant change in the person's status quo. Uncertainty, danger, or even a physical threat may be perceived. The alarm triggers subcortical activation of the autonomic nervous system. Sympathetic nervous system hyperactivity, commonly known as the "fight or flight" response, includes tachycardia, tachypnea, elevated blood pressure, sweating, dryness of the mouth, and pupillary dilatation. When parasympathetic hyperactivity predominates, hypotension, bradycardia, weakness, and fainting are encountered (the "vasovagal reaction"). Hence the practical dictum that bad news should be imparted while the recipient is seated. Furthermore, because of sympathetic and/or parasympathetic hyperactivity, persons receiving tragic news are themselves at greater risk of sudden death.[5]

Anxiety typically appears after alarm. The psychologic signs and symptoms of anxiety become manifest upon comprehension of the full meaning of the news. Persons may react by becoming withdrawn or irritable; they may appear frightened, wring their hands, hyperventilate, or weep. They are aware of the loss of support from the person who has died, and they experience confusion and psychic pain.

Anger follows anxiety. Unconsciously the bereaved is often angry at having been abandoned. The anger may be directed either inward, leading to depression, or outward toward persons in the immediate surroundings. Often the emergency room staff is the target of this anger for imagined shortcomings in the treatment of the deceased. Such reactions may be overtly hostile and occasionally even violent.[6]

More extreme reactions may occur in some persons either as the result of cultural influences or the circumstances in which death occurs. The response of a mother to the death of a young child is often overwhelming. Similarly, deaths that are unexpected or gruesome, such as homicide and suicide, may evoke an exaggerated grief reaction. The reactions encountered may include loud cries, moaning, chanting, and self-abuse.

MANAGEMENT OF THE IMMEDIATE PHASE

General Principles

Persons will remember vividly the circumstances under which they received the news of the death of a loved one. Often they will be able to recall exactly the context, the tone, and the inflection used by the informant. The news preferably should be imparted by the physician who was primarily involved in the care of the patient or by the most senior associate. Otherwise the family may infer that there is a therapeutic misadventure and the physician is ashamed to face them. Alternatively, the family may conclude that the outcome of the treatment of their loved one was unimportant to the physician. The bereaved should first be given an indication that the news that is about to be transmitted is serious, thereby allowing them time to mobilize their defenses. The persons might be prepared with a statement such as "Let's go and sit down in a private room. I need to talk with you." This alerts the listener to prepare for the worst.

It is a good rule to rehearse exactly what is to be said. The news should be presented in a clear and concise manner. Evasiveness and ambiguous terms should be avoided. The family has to know that the patient has died, and they have a need and a right to a statement of the medical facts. Thus, they should be provided with a clear description of the medical course and the type of treatment that was administered. It should be stated that all possible therapeutic efforts were used. The family will be somewhat reassured by the knowledge that the care given was timely and vigorous. An honest summary of the medical emergency should be provided, including an account of the insuperable problems encountered. Families usually want to know the actual cause of death and the suffering endured before death. After the news is given to the family and their questions have been answered, they should be left alone to cry or even scream out their agony without concern for shame or embarrassment.[7]

Special Considerations

There may be one member whom the family will expect to have the most profound reaction to the loss of a loved one. In some situations, one person may take on the role of "chief mourner" and feel obliged to demonstrate feelings for all of the family. Typically, this person is the spouse or mother of the deceased. Not infrequently, rivalries may be present, that is, there may be more than one "chief mourner," and they may compete in demonstrating feelings of grief. These persons must be identified quickly because they will require special attention to protect them from overwhelming emotions. Dealing with them will also serve to indicate to the family that the staff is concerned about their welfare.

Ambiance of the Emergency Room

Maintaining an air of dignity in the emergency room and among the staff is fundamental and essential. The staff should be aware that a grieving family is present and avoid inappropriate behavior such as loud talk, jokes, laughter, and casual irreverent conversation.

Administrative Concerns

A member of the emergency room staff may need to

serve as guide, helper, or liaison worker to the family while they are in the emergency room. It is recommended that the nursing supervisor or charge nurse be assigned this responsibility. This person should determine if the family wishes to view the body and, if so, to make the necessary arrangements. Assistance may also be required to arrange for the disposition of the body of the deceased, including completion of legal documents necessary for the release of the body to the funeral director. Requests for autopsy and/or organ donations should be made only by physicians. The family should not be pressured, but should be informed of the usefulness of such procedures.

Medication

Tranquilizers may not reduce the pain but they may postpone it. On the other hand, total denial of psychopharmacologic support can be shortsighted and inhumane.[8] For the bereaved person in the emergency room who is having marked agitation, the use of hydroxyzine hydrochloride (Vistaril), 50 to 100 mg IM, induces a calming effect. Drug therapy is clearly indicated when the grief reaction is physically disabling. A bedtime hypnotic taken at least until the time of the funeral is reasonable. Because important decisions, including funeral arrangements, must be made, excessive sedation should be avoided. We therefore recommend careful use of benzodiazepines. Oxazepam (15 mg t.i.d.) for example, may be prescribed. Other indications for the use of psychopharmacologic agents have been discussed elsewhere.[9]

Crisis Intervention Programs and Follow-up

Usually families deal with bereavement privately or with the help of clergymen, but the bereaved should be informed about other resources available in the community to help them cope with their emotional crisis (eg. walk-in clinics, community mental health clinics, and crisis-intervention clinics). The family should be told explicitly that they can also return to the emergency room for follow-up care if necessary.

Staff Reaction

Staff members are affected by deaths in the emergency room. Frequent witnessing of bereavement in others may lead to adoption of a veneer of callousness or to an exaggerated sensitivity which reduces functional effectiveness. A psychiatric consultant to the emergency room can facilitate open discussion of feelings about death and the attendant reaction of the staff. This forum will permit persons to ventilate special concerns and deal with specific conflicts concerning death. In a broader perspective, issues relating to stress in the practice of emergency room medicine should be reviewed.

CONCLUSIONS

The reaction to bereavement is unique for every person and family. Nevertheless, the patterns of grief reactions can be anticipated with some reliability. Adroit management of the immediate phase of the grief reaction will provide more empathetic and humane care for those who have suffered a loss and will also serve to maintain staff morale and the uninterrupted operation of the emergency room for other purposes.

References

1. Cassem, N.H. The first three steps beyond the grave. *Acute Grief and the Funeral.* Pine,V.R., Kutscher, A.H., Peretz, D., et al. (eds.). Springfield, Ill.: Charles C. Thomas, 1976, p. 14.

2. Lindemann, E. Symptomatology and management of acute grief. *Am. J. Psychiatry* 101:7-21, 1944.

3. Parkes, C.M. Bereavement and mental illness. Part 2. A classification of bereavement reactions. *Br. J. Med. Psychol.* 38:13-26, 1965.

4. Simos, B.G. *A Time to Grieve.* New York: Family Service Association of America, 1979, pp. 49-59; 103-114.

5. Engel, G.L. Sudden and rapid death during psychological stress, folklore or folk wisdom? *Ann. Intern. Med.* 74:771-782, 1971.

6. Simos, B.G., op. cit.

7. Kübler-Ross, E. On the use of psychopharmacologic agents for the dying patient and the bereaved. *Psychopharmacologic Agents for the Terminally Ill and Bereaved.* Goldberg, I.K., Malitz, S., Kutscher, A.H. (eds). Springfield, Ill.: Charles C. Thomas, 1976, p. 7.

8. Twycross, R.G. Acute Grief: a physician's viewpoint. *Acute Grief and the Funeral.* Pine, V.R., Kutscher, A.H., Peretz, D., et al. (eds.). Springfield, Ill.: Charles C. Thomas, 1976, p. 7.

9. Wiener, A. The use of psychopharmacologic agents in the management of the bereaved. *Psychopharmacological Agents for the Terminally Ill and Bereaved.* Goldberg, I.K., Malitz, S., Kutscher, A.H. (eds.). New York: Columbia University Press, 1973, pp. 249-256.

REFLECTIONS ON MEDICAL EDUCATION

Godfrey S. Getz

The most distinctive change that has affected medicine in the last fifty to sixty years is the extent to which it has drawn strength and nourishment from the basic natural sciences. This nurture seems to be providing forever more rapid expansion and development of new capacities of diagnosis and treatment for a vast array of maladies. The ability to delay death itself calls into question the ends of medicine. The horizon looks even rosier than the immediate past. For example, the prospects are bright for improved organ transplants and organ assists and for helpful intervention even in genetic diseases, which until recently were thought to be beyond the reach of medicine. With this as the rapidly expanding frontier of medicine, the emphasis in the education of medical students has naturally been very strongly on scientific medicine, to help them understand the applications of the natural sciences to the current and anticipated curative and palliative therapies. This orientation is reflected in the requirements for entry into medical school—a year of chemisty, physics, and biological science including laboratory hours.

The successes of modern science have benefited greatly from the deepening understanding of individual organ systems and human functions—so deep in fact that in order to fully understand any one of these systems or functions requires a relatively sharp concentration or specialization. The division of medicine into more and more specialties is a reflection of the pace of our improved understanding and our desire for control over a manageable body of knowledge. We are, at least as individual specialist physicians, learning more and more about less and less. We hope that the patient is best served by the collectivity of the special capacities that are being developed. Clearly, there are some problems with this approach, as the further development of this inquiry will attempt to show.

A major orientation within modern medicine places a high premium on the ability to resolve problems by resorting to hard facts, experimentally verifiable. Emphasis is placed on the mastery of new factual and reductionist information as scientific medicine advances with almost explosive momentum. These facts are usually best interpreted in simple and isolated systems (specialization) leading to the physician's sense of security with a particular body of information and its vagaries. This approach, despite its stunning contributions to biomedical science, has limits especially when applied to complex, interactive systems and organisms. The mastery of a specialized area is in its nature exclusionary, eliminating factors and other systems from consideration, except perhaps when their impact is direct and unavoidable. In many of the prominent medical institutions, clinical scientists, intensively investigating their small corner of the medical universe, represent the preeminent role model of the exemplary practitioner's technique. They reflect the highest value in modern scientific medicine. This is the skill to which our medical faculty aspires and the model that is set before the student. Its contributions are immense, and it is not surprising that it plays so prominent a role in our medical education system.

Like all good things these successes have their costs. These costs all ultimately have their impact on the patient-doctor relationship, which every practicing physician would readily acknowledge to be at the essence of the service to the patient. There is a common sense that this relationship has been deeply eroded. It is widely discussed in all kinds of media. It is frequently discussed by medical students and educators and is very often raised during interviews with prospective medical students, reflecting their desire to set themselves apart from the current image of the profession.

For many decades now, medical care has been centered in the hospital, where charges have been rising at a pace soon to be beyond the capacity of the payers, personal or third-party. These charges, until recently, were seldom mentioned, let alone discussed with medical students in an effort to educate physicians to the economic imperative of medical practice. The era of escalation in charges has now come to an abrupt halt, with government, labor, and the media calling for

action on the cost front. In order to attain cost efficiency, cutbacks in services are inevitable. The striving
toward cost efficiency will surely result in the requirement that patient turnover, both inpatient and outpatient, be accelerated. Such efficiency reduces the
time available for the individual patient-doctor interchange. One has to be concerned that these maneuvers
may not always be in support of the highest reasonable
quality of service. Especially may the service reductions affect the least articulate constituency among the
patient population, the poor and the unemployed. The
busy physician in an outpatient clinic of a hospital sees
many patients—a requirement for the efficient use of
hospital resources—and this barely allows adequate
opportunity for the transfer of directly relevant therapeutic instructions, let alone essential and sometimes
detailed information about the natural course of the
patient's disease or persuasive preventative information about the advantages of the modification of a lifestyle or eating pattern. For the inpatient, yearning for
some communication about his daily progress or developing prospects, how often does the busy physician
have the time to *sit down* by the side of the patient's bed
to clearly demonstrate to the vulnerable patient that he
or she (the physician) has a deep concern for the patient
as person? Some emotional responses of the individual
physician that might obstruct a satisfactory patient-
doctor relationship have recently been discussed.[1]
Although these are undoubtedly important, the wide-
spread sense of a deterioration in patient-doctor relationships suggests that structural factors related to
institutional arrangements or patient expectations are
basic to this situation.

Not only finances have been affected by advancing
medical technology. Other institutional costs are evi-

dent. The centering of medical practice in the hospital has certainly expanded the knowledge and experience of physicians by concentrating a large variety of patients in one place which is also the locus of the multiple technological capacities for diagnosis and treatment. Placing the doctor-patient encounter within a more formal institutional setting has tended to depersonalize the relationship in contrast to the earlier times when doctors more usually made home visits, seeing patients *and* families in an environment more conducive to a relaxed and informative interaction. As diagnosis has depended more on laboratory procedures and computers, patients and doctors have become more estranged from each other. With the increasing specialization, patients have not had a single doctor who managed their care, but multiple physicians who attend to one or other special bodily system. This problem is compounded by the very successes of medicine in sustaining patients with multiple diseases into old age. It is a wonder with this form of medical practice that patients do not feel even more alone and alienated than they do. In such an environment, the patient is inevitably vulnerable and dependent.

It is in relation to terminal disease or chronic incurable illness that problems with the interaction between patient and doctor are most stark. The physician most clearly exhibits his mettle as human being in this context. Prior to the era of modern scientific medicine, the physician had no option but to help chronically ill patients and their families attain comfort and adjustment to their fate. The enormous array of technical competences which scientific medicine has now placed in the hands of the modern physician has had several consequences. He spends much of his time in medical school acquiring the skill and understanding to use these tools. He regards these competences as the essence of his skill as physician. He becomes an activist in the application of these skills. The media and personal experience educate patients to expect technical intervention from the physician. In such an environment, the physician, with all his technical skill at hand, is diminished by the inability to mediate a definitive or favorable outcome. Although some physicians are certainly competent to deal with problems of this sort, it is here that they face difficulties with which so many are unable to cope and for which they are frequently unprepared. The intrinsic or endogenous psychological makeup of the doctor may be at the base of the avoidance or denial reactions that so frequently surface in the face of the medical problem that does not lend itself to the analysis, diagnosis, and definitive treatment for which the modern physician is so emphatically educated. This valued scientific education helps to reinforce the physician's self-image—the compassionate but nevertheless scientific analyst who feels comfortable with the factual and the predictable. The patient's expectations and dependencies, drawn from internal hope and public projections, is sure to further solidify this image that the physician has of himself. To be sure, the physicians's education and professional socialization also emphasizes these values. Perhaps this is partly required to further the physician's necessary emotional distance from his or her patients' serious troubles. But this emphasis is built on the natural tendency of all people to feel most comfortable with the known and the predictable. None of us feel comfortable dealing with the unknown, the unpredictable, the ambiguous, especially when the only thing that can be predicted about the situation is that the ultimate outcome will be unfavorable. The challenge of the unexpected, the ambiguous, can be invigorating only when an exciting and profoundly successful end may lie in wait. In the patient with the incurable chronic disease or the terminally ill patient for whom only palliation can be offered, the daily living is uncertain, unpredictable, especially when uninformed by the medical advisor who has the knowledge about the natural course of the illness. These uncertainties can best be tolerated when the patient is secure about his place within his family and his immediate community, and about the concern and devotion to his welfare by his medical advisor. The physician has as one of his major responsibilities the attempt to help sustain this feeling of belonging, which requires that the patient and the family be thoroughly informed about what lies in store for them wherever possible and that the whole unit be secure that the devotion of the physician and medical team can be depended upon.

"There are incurable conditions, but never untreatable patients. Concretely this means that the physician is obliged to learn and advise about ways of living better with illness, through means not generally thought to be medical—involving advice about improved and more encouraging living situations, family support, alternative employment, transportation, etc. It also carries a strong presumption in favor of truthfulness, for the patient's dignity in facing his situation depends on knowing what it is and means.... When one professes medicine, one offers the healing, comforting, and encouraging hand which, when it is grasped, may not be pulled away, at least not without providing for its replacement."[2]

Although the problems with the patient-doctor relationship are generally recognized, the present mode of medical practice is accepted, because of its obvious suc-

cesses in providing definitive therapies and acknowledged, favorable outcomes for so many discomforts
and life-threatening situations. Complaints about the
doctor-patient relationship were early countered by
offering the straw choice between the physician competent to handle and apply the modern medical technology to the patient's benefit and the physician who had
an exemplary "bedside manner" that comforted the
patient without adequately treating his medical problem. This non-choice was offered in justification of the
heavy emphasis given to biomedical science in the
medical curriculum.

A great deal has been written about the compassionate and humane physician. Most physicians probably
are compassionate and humane, even those who are
sometimes accused of being otherwise, but within the
limits of a very comfortable view of their skills in medicine. What they manifest is an inability to deal with the
ambiguity of a personal transaction which cannot be
defined—which has unexpected twists, which foretells
tragic consequences for which no simple remedies are
at hand. We all are most comfortable when we understand our skills, have an ability to use them, and put
them to use in the service of others. Similarly, we feel
comfortable with personal relationships whose course
is predictable with knowing responses on our part. Is
this not why we habitually associate with others of
similar interests, often similar temperament, and similar culture? There is little ambiguity in the relationships of happy partners or happy parents and children.
What happens with relationships in which the predictability of response is questioned? Only the healthiest
relationships can survive this ambiguity.

Although this is a value which is somehow contradictory to those epitomized by the highly successful

biomedical scientist, a good physician needs to be able to tolerate ambiguity—to confront it in his relationships and to deal with it in his personal patient encounters. Perhaps then he will not retreat from his chronically ill patient, for whom he cannot prescribe the definitive therapy, or from the dying patient, who cannot be restored to even temporary health by the miracles of modern medicine. In supporting his patient and tending to his needs, he has to be able to face the unpredictable unravelling of family and personal tensions. If only he will forget the unrealistic expectations with which he has been anointed by society and the projections of his colleagues and carry with him the naturally decent and compassionate inclinations which led him into medicine, he will discharge these obligations admirably. "...There were so many people needing help, and so little that he could do for any of them. It was necessary for him to be available, and to make all these calls at their homes, but I was not to have the idea that he could do anything much to change the course of their illness."[3]

Many prescriptions for the education of the caring physician have been offered. I will not desist from offering mine. It has three parts. First, at the premedical level, I advocate that students be required to take a year of literature, a year of social science and a year of a subject devoted to an historical perspective. When combined with a year of chemistry, physics, and biology this may seem a tall order. Perhaps, but it is after all simply a well-rounded liberal education and no more than is expected of any natural science major at the University of Chicago. In addition to being a liberal education, which is its highest attribute, it can be justified as a self-conscious and significant contribution to the professional background of the physician. It has been correctly claimed that you cannot make a caring and humane physician by asking him to take courses. Perhaps so, but challenging courses can heighten already-existing sensitivities and instincts of compassion which, in the medical education arena, are taken for granted and are frequently not explicitly reinforced by shared discussion of students and faculty. A similar suggestion is put forward in two thoughtful articles in *Pharos* (Summer 1983).[4],[5]

It makes little matter precisely what literature is studied as long as it is good—classic works. Classic works of art, literature, and poetry all possess sufficient ambiguity that each new approach to such a work reveals new insights that relate to the particular responsiveness of the viewer or reader. Classic works of literature frequently represent distillations of general wisdom and insight, teaching us to understand the complexities of human nature and human relationships. This study would represent a counterweight to the hard science so emphatically focused upon, and help students to appreciate the natural and the wise, to understand the meaning of myth and symbol that can be so valuable in dealing with those persons from a different cultural background than oneself. Good literature could reveal for us the difficulty of human nature, the subtleties of human communication, and help us to remain above the short-term expressions of hostility that may intrude on the patient-doctor relationship. But most of all, the study of great literature could help us to view the world with an easier tolerance of the ambiguous. There can be few more striking examples of the felicitous amalgam of science and literature than Sir William Osler. It was his practice to end the day with an hour of reading—never medical. If he chanced upon a colleague reading a textbook in bed, he would go to his library, find a classic and hand it to the surprised friend. "Here, this is more worthwhile."[6]

With social science, it is important to learn about the relationships between communities and institutions, to understand what societal forces help to form public policy and community morality so that the place of the medical profession and its patients may be appreciated in the broader scheme of things. The cultural diversity of different human communities and their behaviors would be explored in most general sequences in the social sciences. Insights gained from such studies may help students and graduates to understand the complex social and psychological forces that condition the "addicts," alcoholics, and recidivist patients for whom it is so easy to develop a distaste.

The historical orientation is included to ensure that students develop a long view of the evolution of ideas and learn that humility is appropriate in relation to the commonly held ideas in science and human relationships.

Although many students probably already undertake a program similar to that outlined above, its declaration as requirement for entry into medical school would probably stimulate the student to a self-conscious reflection on the impact of liberal studies for the broadminded practice of medicine.

Secondly, devices need to be found to sustain the genuine sensitivity and humaneness with which most medical students enter medical school. It is acknowledged that a certain level of detachment and emotional distance is necessary to enable physicians to deal with the panoply of human suffering that constitutes the experience of the average physician. This is achieved through the learning of a new technical language that tends to remove the emotional content from a description of human suffering and through other forms of socialization acquired from the faculty models to whom students are exposed. But, on the other hand, the patient needs to feel that the doctor is devoted to his general welfare. The development of a proper balance between these two counterweights needs to be explicitly dealt with through student and faculty discussion and support groups. Otherwise, there is a great risk that the maturing student will acquire his or her attitudes from faculty who, in the student's experience, seem to have the most status in the institution and not necessarily the best balance between technical competence, professionalism, and humane behavior towards patients. In some places attempts are being made to address this issue directly in the clinical curriculum.[7]

Finally, the development of attitudes and skills in dealing with the chronically ill and terminally sick is one of the most challenging needs in the education of physicians. The ability to provide advice about "ways of living better" requires an understanding of the patient's family and social relationships, the patient's ability to adapt to a work situation and to cope with his daily living environment. It is difficult to acquire this knowledge of the patient when he or she is seen mainly and perhaps exclusively in the institutional setting. Furthermore, although Gorlin and Zucker (1983) are attempting to deal with this problem in the traditional institutional setting, mainly by having residents function essentially as family physicians, it is difficult to see this phase of the student's education being completed within the boundaries of the traditional medical school. These are mostly based in tertiary care hospitals, where some or all of the teaching is done by medical specialists and clinical scientists who have major demands on their time other than for clinical care.

Many of them have substantial university administrative responsibilities, necessary departmental obligations, active research time demands, administrative and scientific responsibilities that extend outside the medical school, all perfectly appropriate. But *time with the patient* is essential to meet the criteria of the "compleat" physician, and this is a commodity which is in very short supply among the senior visible physicians who have the wisdom and experience to be most helpful in this phase of a student's education. It is *time with the patient* that is eroded by the physician's other responsibilities, his need to teach, do research, keep abreast of the advancing frontiers of medicine, and by the drive toward cost efficiency, as well as the organization of hospital practice. Dealing with the problem posed here is not easy, and no ready prescription comes to mind. Many medical students have elective time in the senior year, and often, this time is employed off campus. Perhaps students should be encouraged, if not required, to spend this time in work away from the traditional tertiary care center, with family practitioners, with a hospice, or in quite other institutional settings. Among the more radical suggestions is that of Stetten, who believes that students should experience the handicaps of simulated blindness or a broken limb.[8] Clearly, further experimentation is required to meet this challenge in student education.

It is clear that modern medical practice presents a paradox—tension between the display of technical and scientific skill and the attention to the personal needs of the patient. The challenge of the physician, the educator, and the student is to attain the proper balance in this productive tension—to practice in proper measure the art and science of medicine.

ACKNOWLEDGEMENT

I am indebted to Daniel Segal, whose study in medical education, "The Routines of Charisma" (M.A. Thesis, Department of Anthropology, University of Chicago), was most instructive, approaching his field work with freshness and tolerance.

It is a great pleasure to acknowledge the contributions of Drs. Pauline and David Rabin, whose fortitude, candor and pertinacity, and stimulating and encouraging discussions were really responsible for me writing this essay.

References

1. Gorlin, R. and Zucker, H.D. Physician's reactions to patients. A key to teaching humanistic medicine. *N. Engl. J. Med.* 308:1059-1063, 1983.

2. Kass, L.R. Professing ethically. On the place of ethics in defining medicine. *J.A.M.A.* 249:1305-1310, 1983.

3. Thomas, L. *The Youngest Science: Notes of a Medicine-Watcher.* New York: The Viking Press, 1983.

4. Dugan, N.L. The professionalization of feeling (editorial). *Pharos* 46:41, 1983 (summer).

5. Stetten, D.J. Tomorrow's physician. *Pharos* 46:26, 1983 (summer).

6. Cushing, H. *The Life of Sir William Osler*. Oxford at the Clarendon Press, 1925.

7. Gorlin and Zucker, op. cit.

8. Stetten, D.J., op. cit.

SOME REFLECTIONS ON HUMANISM IN MEDICINE

Roscoe R. Robinson and F. Tremaine Billings

There is an increasing concern, in this country and elsewhere, that today's doctors are somewhat lacking in their display of the human qualities so long associated with the image of a true physician. Observers within and without the medical profession, including our patients, acknowledge that we are tending to the bodies of the sick with increasing effectiveness, but they find us wanting in our commitment to comfort and help their souls. Caring, compassion, empathy, understanding, and responsiveness to the human needs of patients are felt to be less evident than was the case in earlier times, and those of us in medical education are urged to renew and strengthen our emphasis on the necessity of such qualities in our students.

Such concerns are not new. The proper conduct of physicians, or the lack thereof, has been a subject of frequent discourse of hundreds of years. Throughout, the peoples of various societies have voiced a strong and steadfast plea for humanistic behavior on the part of those who were chosen or permitted to care for their illnesses. The expressions of earlier observers suggest that the gap between the public perception of the humanistic attributes of its physicians and its expectation has never been closed completely. In explanation of this shortfall, it is tempting for physicians to take easy refuge in the possibility that public expectations of its doctors have always been too high. Instead, it is our responsibility first to consider other reasons why the gap has not been closed, and ask repeatedly to what extent the fault may be ours alone. Toward that end, there is today a growing view that the gap has become uncomfortably wide, that there is too little compassion in the treatment of our patients, that we can certainly do better than we are doing now, and that we must somehow encourage a reaffirmation of the importance of humanistic qualities among physicians. What are the circumstances that have given rise to these views, and how can they be best addressed?

As we set about to consider the above issues, one of us (F.T.B.) volunteered to take the first important step and prepare a rough draft for future discussion and editing. Upon review of that initial effort, it was agreed that the flavor of a number of issues had been so caught that its unedited reproduction was justified:

> The day of sophisticated and revealing high technology is upon us. Magic procedures and drugs for the diagnosis and treatment of complicated diseases—cancer, heart attacks—are at hand.

We are obsessed by them. We are hypnotized by them.

We feel compelled to use them all—exciting new technology and magic drugs—because they are here. We can now diagnose disease without speaking to or even touching patients and we can keep them alive indefinitely despite themselves and sometimes without regard to their wishes.

Adding to the excitement and the tantalizing aura of the above situation is the emergence of the team concept of patient care. Things have gotten too complicated for a single doctor to understand what's going on. So, for each organ to be examined, for each disease to be diagnosed and treated, a specialist is called to the scene.

The viewer of scans, the listener to echoes, the student of bone marrows, the chemotherapeutic medicine man, the endoscopist, the catheterizer of hearts—"to each his own."

For understanding and help with his or her own practice or personal problems, the patient is sometimes left confused. It is even possible that in the beginning a caring, listening, empathetic history and physical examination will have been omitted. The machines and laboratory tests will tell us what we want to know with more specificity and less subjectivity. Personal feelings and basic questions such as "Why doesn't my body function?" "Why do I feel so badly?" "Why am I nauseated?" "Why am I tired?" and "Why do I feel old?" are ping-ponged back and forth between specialist, ricocheting here and there and falling through the cracks.

The physician who listens to the patient, who cares for and guides the family, who brings the parts together, in short, the doctor who deals with the whole person, is said to be less evident. Communication between consultants and the referring physician may be tenuous. It becomes even more tenuous during the prolonged course of a complicated illness as the need for closer communication and support grows.

A thorough and continuing understanding of the ever-growing and expanding body of knowledge of human physiology and pathology is absolutely essential. A full comprehension of the capabilities and uses of newly available technology must be grasped. Principles for the use of an enlarging array of drugs, now delicately and specifically useful for the treatment of many types of disease such as cardiac, cancer, infectious, renal, must be learned and updated constantly. A strong scientific base and a constantly continuing scientific education are vital. It is well known that a humanistic and outdated physician can lead his or her patient to death. The specialized investigation and treatment of disease is here to stay, even as we know that most of these dramatic and successful additions to our armamentarium can be the cause of serious and potentially fatal side-effects.

So what do we expect in a physician? Perhaps we expect an impossible combination of characteristics. Dr. James B. Herrick, one hundred years ago, put it well when he said the physician should have a dual personality, i.e., he or she should be "scientific toward the disease but human toward the patient." At risk of being called "chauvinistic internists," we might ask whether a urologist or a dermatologist, who is expert in genito-urinary function or diseases of the skin, can or should be expected to involve himself in a patient's combined psychological and physical problems. The answer is simple: all physicians must be interested and they should try.

In our effort to expose the medical student and young house-officer to a flood of potentially overwhelming and ever-growing scientific data, we run a great risk of overlooking the nonscientific, ever-present, and growing problems of people. We have carefully selected students for medicine who are strong in science. Have those with humanistic traits been selected with equal care? The answer is probably "No." Scientific strength and cognitive performance can be measured by grades and scores. Compassion, empathy, and enjoyment of people, the art of listening, and a warm receptive nature cannot be measured nearly as well. Such characteristics are usually conceived in childhood and further developed at mother's knee. We must search for them and encourage their growth in our students and young physicians. Explosive progress in the treatment of hitherto deadly diseases, and the excitement engendered by the arrest or cure of otherwise fatal cancer, may have distorted the view of our own powers and kindled an unrealistic feeling of accomplishment. Serious decisions are being made regarding living and dying, and such decisions are now much more complicated for both the patient and the physician. Too frequent, the battle is waged between the physician and the disease with insufficient consideration of the patient's overall or long-term welfare. The patient is caught between two unrelenting forces.

In this sometimes lonely world of intensive and disease-oriented investigation and management, there is the greatest need for a scientifically based physician who is also people-oriented and interested in caring for the patient as a whole.

Several major concerns are addressed in the first draft 1) the arrival of advanced technology and an explosive growth of scientific knowledge may have diverted our attention from the need to comfort those who suffer; 2) the need for greater humanism must not be met at the expense of a lessened commitment to the facts and science of medicine; 3) the individual sense of responsibility for the welfare of a patient can be diffused unduly by the process of team care; 4) the importance and necessity of adequate doctor-doctor and doctor-patient communication cannot be emphasized too strongly; 5) our patients and the public may have come to expect too much; 6) we must search for better ways to identify, develop, nurture and reward the traits of humanism in physicians.

Let us consider a few selected facets of these concerns

further, while touching briefly on others along the way.

First, if greater humanism is to be encouraged among our students and young physicians in training, we must be clear as to the nature of those qualities that are perhaps most essential to the humane physician. It is our view that there are four: compassion, honesty, a reasonable understanding of one's self, and an appreciation of the rights of those under our care.

The acquisition of a personal quality such as compassion is not taught easily, if it can be taught at all. Medical school faculties have yet to define a satisfactory course in "Compassionate Medicine 101" for students as they prepare to approach the wards. Instead, we must rely on role-modeling as the most effective means of transmitting the importance of compassion and the other ingredients of humanism to our students. But the role-modeling of humanism is doomed to failure unless it is practiced daily by a majority of the faculty. Students must learn to recognize and comment on its absence in their mentors. Its importance must be driven home to students by evidence of an institutional commitment to science *and* humanism. Appropriate and meaningful rewards must be devised for those who practice a caring attitude, but only if they also display a requisite knowledge of biomedical science and human diseases. Compassion alone does not make a doctor. Faculty must teach by example without fear of acknowledging that they may not always do it right or well. Students should be encouraged to ask their teachers to explain the rationale for their behavior with patients, just as they might ask them to explain the pathophysiology of chronic renal failure.

Compassion must be accompanied by an urge to help and by an active personal participation in the problems of a patient, not only by an intellectual commitment, but also by an emotional one. This quality, this deep involvement, must be inclusive of all those who put their trust in us. It cannot only include the influential, bright and shiny, compliant carriage trade whose association with us can give us prestige and make us feel important. Our compassion must especially reach out to embrace the poor, downtrodden, and underprivileged who come to us with insuperable personal, socioeconomic, psychologic, and organic problems. Here is where the challenge lies. Here is the opportunity to help those who cannot help themselves.

Self-evaluation as one approaches a career in medicine is unusually important. It is particularly necessary to determine one's motives early. The profession of medicine has a wide variety of facets wherein one may find satisfaction and productivity: there is the excitement and challenge of scientific research broadening the horizons of knowledge; there is the inspiring experience of teaching and the opportunity to stimulate others; and there is the broadly based satisfaction of caring for patients. These are the three major driving forces of medicine and fortunate is the physician who can successfully be involved in all three. There are, of course, other influences which may motivate a young person to go into medicine, and to these following reasons one must be wary: social and community prestige and financial reward. Medicine is an honorable profession and, if pursued honestly and conscientiously, will bring its own reward. But as the cost of health care in general has escalated the reputation of the physician in particular as a greedy overcharger has emerged. How many operations does it take to buy a brand-new sports car and the biggest house on the hill? The practice of medicine has always provided a comfortable, respectable living. Let that be the goal. Remember, were it not for their patients' illnesses and misfortunes doctors would starve.

Young physicians must place the highest value on an honest self-appraisal of their own skills and abilities. Few failings of a physician are worse than the inability, through either ignorance or prideful reluctance, to acknowledge the limits of his or her own knowledge or expertise. No doctor's therapeutic armamentarium is complete unless it includes a highly developed sensitivity and brisk responsiveness to the possible need for consultation or referral. Conversely, it is a reflection of false pride and a form of dishonesty that wishes to divert or take offense at a patient's request for a second professional opinion. Patients extend a special trust when they choose a doctor, a fact that is not honored completely unless the acceptance of that trust is coupled with an equally special form of honesty with one's self, a faithfulness to one's promises to the patient, and the two-way maintenance of communication.

We are still impressed by the remarkable tolerance of patients to unavoidable delay or other inconveniences in the course of a visit to their doctor if and when someone has taken the time to explain their cause courteously, and if and when it is perceived by them that their care and their physician are of the highest quality. Many misunderstandings between doctors and their patients, including not a few malpractice suits, could be avoided if the doctor only took the time to comfort the patient, or tend to his or her sorrow, to counsel warmly, and to explain the nature of the poorly understood events that almost always surround the evaluation or treatment of any illness. Communication, through spoken language or facial expression, is perhaps the single most important ingredient in the effective practice of the "art" of medicine. Its development and use deserve a measure of care and attention equivalent to that required for the acquisition and usage of other procedural skills. And as we talk to our patients, we must still remember that sick people are not normal people. Permanent judgment of any patient's character or personality can only be reserved when that person is seen only in the midst of sickness and suffering. Reservation of that judgment does not come easily when the doctor has been exposed to anger, frustration, or abuse. Lastly, communication with our patients is supposed to be bidirectional. Most especially, we should listen to what our patients have to say about us and other doctors. We can learn from them.

We must develop a sense of self-understanding if we are to recognize and control our own instinctive responses to insult, abuse, anger, intolerance, aggression, or other forms of unattractive behavior by our patients. Such behavior would be equally unattractive in us. We must recognize that there is little time or room for dogmatism, arrogance, or prideful egocentricity on our part, except on network television. The world around *us* does not move. Certainly, repulsion and anger in response to unacceptable behavior, and even a dislike of one's patient, can be normal human responses. But effective doctoring is best carried out if such reactions and their origins are recognized as they appear, so that we can ask ourselves objectively if their appearance has interfered, or threatens to interfere, with care of the patient.

It is important to realize that all patients will not react as we wish. Some are disagreeable and demanding and even critical of us. Some even have problems which cannot be scientifically explained. They may complain as though they had organic illnesses and can be altogether unattractive. Even more disconcerting are patients who won't get well, who won't respond to our most conscientious efforts and ministration, and whose illnesses we discover are inexorably ongoing either because we know that that is the nature of the disorder or because we do not understand it.

Under all these conditions the physician feels that he or she has failed, and unless very careful, is inclined to pass the blame of the failure on to the patient. That, of course, will never do. This is a time for careful self-evaluation and an effort for self-understanding. One must realize that if things are not going well for the doctor, they must be going worse for the patient. Renewed warm, steady, supportive attention to and communication with the patient are, therefore, especially important.

We should ask more frequently if our decisions on the style and manner of our practices are made with the patient's interests first in mind, or our own. A busy and demanding schedule can be used too easily as an excuse for patterns of practice that are designed exclusively for the convenience of the doctor rather than the patient. The doctor whose hospital rounds can only be held late at night (when visiting hours are over) is not only inconsiderate of the needs of patients and their families, but guilty of sending a strong signal that his or her convenience is far more important than that of the patient.

Even much more important than this is the need for careful understanding that it is the patient's and responsible family's right, and theirs alone, to make final decisions regarding treatment, lifestyle, dignity, and matters of life and death. These decisions must be made in careful concert and in completely supportive communication with the responsible physician who has gathered and made available all the complicated information from various investigative procedures and consultants. This communication must be ongoing, complete, and continuously up-to-date. Advice and guidance can and should be offered, but the patient and family must be fully informed and encouraged to make final decisions. No longer can we say, "Don't ask questions, trust me." Patients and families know many answers and only trust doctors when fully informed.

What can we do as faculty to encourage the development of positive human qualities in our students? Are certain training experiences to be avoided, modified, or discontinued? Answers to such questions do not come quickly or completely, but search for them we must.

The central importance of role-modeling has already been discussed. Specialist or not, our clinical teachers should be required to concern themselves with the whole patient, including the quality of his or her life and human needs, and to do it every day. We must consider the impact of advanced technology and treatment on our patients and learn to work more effectively with nurses and others who care. The art of communication and talking with our patients and each other must be emphasized, as must a structured opportunity for continuity of patient care in the hospital, the doctor's office, and the home. We must make ourselves available to our students and demonstrate our concern for the patient at the bedside, and not within the recess of a distant conference room. We must place more emphasis on careful understanding of patients and their illnesses and thus place some constraint on the excessive use of costly diagnostic procedures. Our teaching rounds must convey a feeling of responsibility for the outcome of a recommended approach to the evaluation of a patient's problems and a consideration for the inconveniences and, indeed, possible dangers to the patient which may accompany such an approach. Our preoccupation with knowing the "facts" must be extended to include the human needs of sick people. The recognition of humanism, and appropriate awards therefore, should be included in our evaluation of students just as we now evaluate and reward those who have addressed the science of medicine satisfactorily. As much as anything, humanism is an attitude and its application is fostered best by constant and visible commitment to its precepts. Exposure to structured conferences in ethics and related topics can be provided, but we have to prove to our students that humane approaches to health care do make a difference in clinical outcomes. Facets of our training programs are intended properly to be rigorous, busy, and demanding, but consistent overwork and excessive fatigue can no longer be condoned.

Whatever our approach, it is up to us to respond to those who claim that we are insensitive to the human needs of our patients, that we are arrogant, and that we are excessively preoccupied with science, laboratory tests, and advanced technology. We must recognize that our curricular emphases, while perhaps reflecting an effective means of transmitting the science of medicine, may be less effective in their transmission of the art and humanity of medicine.

Therein lies the challenge. It was perhaps recognized in 1925 by Canby Robinson, the first Dean of the new Vanderbilt University School of Medicine, when he said: "The severest criticism against modern medical education is perhaps directed at its lack of success in teaching the art of medicine." We, the faculty, must reaffirm our commitment to teaching the art and humanity of medicine, on the wards and at the bedside of the patient. And as we so do, we must remember, always, that there still remain those intangible attributes of head and heart that make the true physician, and that such attributes can only be developed at our side and in the common environment of a caring, attractive, and well-run ward or clinic.

A PHILOSOPHER REFLECTS: A PLAY AGAINST NIGHT'S ADVANCE

Richard M. Zaner

What follows here has been quite difficult to write. Not, as I might have initially thought, because of the possible affront to David and Pauline Rabin an article on being ill may have been. What made this thing hard was a comment David Rabin made in response to something I had written about that topic some time earlier, focusing on end-stage renal disease and hemodialysis.[1] In fact, his comment stunned me: everything I then tried to write seemed somehow irreverent and irrelevant. Since my pursuit of that subtly fugitive idea seems part of the thing, I've decided that there is nothing for it but to record at least something of my course, my efforts to track it down.

In that earlier essay, I was struck by the pervasiveness of sheer chance and contingency in human life. Try as we will, we often seem unable to make good sense of so many of the plain accidents which are definitive of what and who we are. I was led to note how deeply this marks the experience of illness and injury ("accidents," both!). Patients suffering from end-stage renal failure and on the grueling nutritional and medical regimens requisite to maintain them until the chance for transplantation comes about, or else death overtakes, exhibit a profound sense of this contingency, of what Pascal once called the "infinity of chance happening...a thousand unforeseen things."[2] The experience of illness or injury has a common thematic metaphor: "How the hell did I get here?"[3]

That theme, poignant and with its own inevitable sense of the tragic, is nevertheless but an indication of the truly radical contingency which marks our very existence. As Herbert Speigelberg has suggested in a series of wonderfully insightful and historically informed articles,[4,5,6,7,8] "it is chance in a specific and very definite sense which is ultimately responsible for all we initally are and have." In this sense, being born (as "human," as "me," or even being born at all) is an "accident": an act done to us and over which we had neither control nor knowledge, and which was neither chosen nor deserved. Moreover, "prior to any conscious action or choice of our own we find ourselves already born into stations and into their inequalities. They are, as it were, thrown upon us, certainly without any consciousness of having deserved them. Nor is there any objective evidence that they depend upon any moral desert. This lack of a moral title and primarily of a moral desert for our initial shares in life I...call here 'moral chance.' "[9] It was this theme, and the ethical responsibility it seems to entail—namely, as our accidents of birth are unwarranted, advantages and handicaps alike, the inequalities of birth call for redress, moral equalization—which preoccupied me in that essay.

One thing those reflections made prominent was the other side of our congenital lot or fate: "luck," whether "good" or "bad." Watching a heretic being led to execution, John Bradford exclaimed: "There, but for the grace of God, go I!" Some of us are fortunate, were born into good, loving families, endowed with good health, and blessed with talent and with nurturing friends and surroundings. Others of us are not so "lucky."

Albert Schweitzer, apparently alone and utterly original in this, came to his "other thought"—other than his profound reverence for life—in precisely this context. Having been born into a well-situated and loving family, with immense talent and sound physical health, he yet believed that "I must not accept this good fortune as a matter of course but had to give something in return."[10] Neither "good fortune" nor congenital handicaps are deserved; both are equally unjust in the specific sense of having been due to "moral chance," something done to us without choice or desert.

Thus, Schweitzer urged that "no one has the right to take for granted his own advantages over others in health, talents, in ability, in success, in a happy childhood, and congenial home conditions. One must pay the price for all these boons. What we owe in return is a special responsibility for other lives," especially those with no less undeserved and unchosen burdens, disadvantages, and handicaps.[11]

Those of us less fortunate, seemingly victims and pawns of outrageous fortune, may be understandably led to profound bewilderment, rage, and despair at the sheer capriciousness of our lots: "Why me?" and "Just when things had finally begun to work..." are typical of our sense of the unearned fates we suffer. Something, we believe, is profoundly unjust about a world in which, by the sheerest of accidents and wholly undeserved, debilitating illness or injury is visited on us—often just when it is least wanted and most hurtful.

"Arterio—what was that you said?"

"—sclerosis."

"Bunky?"

"*Our* Bunky?"

"Yes."

"God!"

"*Sic transit gloria mundi.* A rare case. Poor chap—went out like a light. Just like a light."

"But I mean—Bunky, of all people! Up in his studies, young, well-off, good-looking, everything to live for!"

"*Ave atque vale*, old boy."

"I can't believe it."

"Here today, gone tomorrow."

"God!"

Here, in the opening scene of Charles Beaumont's short story "Hair of the Dog,"[12] it is painfully clear that illness, disaster, misfortune are *never* timely, *never* fitting, *never* comprehensible. None of the daily platitudes effectively grips the thing, makes it understandable. "Why Bunky?" "Why me?" And the nudge of the only response is chilling: there simply *is* no reason, good or otherwise; rather, "That's the way the ball bounces," "That's just one of those things," "*Sic transit gloria mundi*," "Here today, gone tomorrow." But neither the caprice of the occurrence nor the platitudes responding to the accidents comfort or explain.

And now, I can say what stunned me when I first met David Rabin and we chatted—or, rather, I talked, he nodded and listened, eyes alert and acute, and every so often, with Pauline's help, and with great effort, he uttered his words as much as the tracheotomy permitted. His words? Pauline had to interpret them for me. They concerned the "Why me?" and he said, haltingly but oh, so pointedly: "Why *not* me?" Why *not*?

It wasn't until I had left, returned home, and was thinking about our talk, when it hit. Had I heard correctly? Here was David Rabin, in the full ravages of ALS—paralyzed in every way save for facial and some neck muscles, tracheotomy in place, labored breathing needing periodic suctioning, unable to talk except in short gasps, yet keenly alert in mind and eye. "Why *not* me?" That seems the luxury of the very healthy, the comfortable, easy words of abstract and painless life snug in its complacent niche of health and normalcy. To such persons it is easy to say such words: easy to say, horribly hard to live through. But David spoke them.

I can't suppose my silence at the time was from shock, not even from self-denial, nor even politeness. Candidly, I passed it over (it passed me by) in the way such things do in a usual sort of conversation.

Only afterward did it dawn on me, when I sat down to write my contribution to this volume. My contribution which was to have been a further probing of the caprice lying within human life, especially on occasions of confronting illness. It could still be that, but David Rabin's response keeps insinuating itself, even though its point remains obscure. Yet, what he said and the context in which it was said seem somehow significant. So I've decided to pursue it; or, rather, to see whether I am able to allow this elusive theme to emerge honestly.

A perhaps circuitous route occurs to me: maybe David Rabin was joshing me a bit, engaging in a bit of ironic play like Ben Harrison in the movie *Whose Life Is It Anyway*? "Why me?" "Well, why not?" As Pauline translated and interpreted for me, however, he was not simply playing with words or ideas: David's experience, brought to the fore when he read my article, was never the "Why me?" sort. It was rather the "Why not me?" So, if there was a bit of by-play going on, it was also most serious play.

But can these two ideas be thought together: play and seriousness? Of course they can. People, and not only children, can be at times deadly serious about play, to the point of deadening boorishness. But that observation doesn't help; the thing changes when it is a matter of a person so grievously afflicted as David Rabin. Here, there simply is no room for play, by-play, playfulness, or the rest. Illness, I will be quickly reminded, is serious business: how much joviality does one find in a hospital, in the room of a dying person, or in the presence of an ALS victim in the final stages of that dreadful disease? And, when it is a matter of playing around with grievous illness, or with death, humor seems little short of obscene.

And yet, the fact which set me thinking was not anything I said or felt, but to the contrary what he said. Does it make any sense for a person struck down by that dread disease, paralyzed and debilitated in almost every way except in mental alertness, without having deserved it, and knowing that nothing can be done to stay its fateful course—does it make any sense for *this* man to say, "Why *not* me?"

I confess: when I later thought about that scene, I smiled; right now, as I recall it, I have to laugh, for he caught me short and up-ended my altogether ponderous seriousness. There is something at once quite simple yet subtly elusive here. I want to try to say it, but like all things subtle and magical the only way to get at it is by a kind of indirection. My way concerns how we typically understand play and culture, and what's wrong with that?

What is this common, received understanding? Consider, first, the phenomenon of play. Where there is play, we are told, games are soon to come: the first prepares the way for and gradually becomes transformed into the other, as children grow into adulthood. This transformation is another name for socialization. As the child grows up, Piaget[13] and Mead[14] argue, there is an increase of rule-governed activity and, with that, an increase of *work* over play. The "seriousness of life," work, overtakes the easy spontaneity of childhood's play. As children become adults, the predominant forms of play are games, "socialized games, controlled by rules,"[15] and childhood playfulness ("childishness") diminishes, to be absorbed into the prevailing web of rules, roles, and codes both written and unwritten which characterize adult life. Eventually, social conduct is governed by what Mead calls "the generalized Other": the awareness of "the team," the "rules of the game," "the community," "the law," and "society" more generally.[16] A person who persists in "play" is a person who has not yet "grown up" or "matured."

Such a view of play and work conforms closely to the received paradigm of the nature of social life. Peter Berger, along with and on the basis of the work of Alfred Schutz, has with rare intelligence given some of the more significant insights into the workings of the social order, especially in his marvelous book *The Sacred Canopy*.[17] To live in a social world is to live an ordered and meaningful life, in the embrace of an overarching "social nomos" (order, rule, law). Human culture, constructed within the imposed limits of human biology, provides the "firm structures for human life that are lacking biologically," such as institutions for marriage, child-rearing, education, commerce, and the like. Yet, although culture is inherently unstable and subject to change, it tends toward stability, temporal endurance, and objectivity. While each individual contributes to and sustains the prevailing culture, each is at the same time deeply enculturated and socialized.

Culture outlasts each individual, even while each contributes to culture. The paradigmatic case of this tensioned relation is that of language, the common tongue. We are unable to speak meaningfully except by means of the culturally imposed language, yet in any individual's usage of the language it is both subtly changed and sustained in its objective existence.

We "take on" social roles as we grow older, and thereby also take on a complex cluster of attitudes, beliefs, conducts, and values. We "internalize" these and thereby also "identify" with them. Thus, each of us is not only deeply socialized into the ways and byways of culture, but we also represent and express these attitudes and values in every form of conduct. Thus, from the "uncultured" innocence of childhood's play, human development is said to mature into socialized roles, codes, rules, and laws defining what it is to be a legitimate, adult member of that culture.

The fuller story is, of course, much more complex. Enough is at hand for it to be recognized how this standard view of culture and society views, indeed *must* view, any serious rupture of that nurturing fabric or order. Such a break with the expected routines and values of social life, Berger contends, is at the very least "a powerful threat" both to the individual and to the social order. The more serious the breech, the greater the loss of deeply satisfying emotional and valuational bonds. More than that, the individual is threatened by a loss of bearings, of orientation in life. "In extreme cases," Berger writes, "he loses his sense of reality and identity. He becomes anomic (i.e. without order) in the sense of becoming worldless." While the circumstances of such "nomic disruption" may vary for different persons, its significance is nonetheless that the person will "lose his moral bearings, with disastrous psychological consequences." He will become cognitively shattered, in the sense that he is no longer capable of reckoning with things "as they are."

The social order is "a shield against terror." Since people "are congenitally compelled to impose a meaningful order upon reality...the ultimate danger of such a separation...is the danger of meaninglessness." Accordingly, the received view of social reality is committed to the idea that the "nightmare *par excellence*" is the breech of the social order (i.e. anomy), and submerges the individuals suffering that break "in a world of disorder, senselessness, and madness."

The sheltering quality of, and the threat of a breech in, the prevailing social order seems no more apparent than in what Karl Jaspers calls "marginal" or "limiting" situations (Grenzsituations).[18] These are situations in which a person is driven to or close to the boundaries of the order determining social life itself. For Jaspers, the extreme is the encounter with one's own death. But any situation in which that is disclosed or hinted at—e.g. illness, injury, loss, danger—is one which inherently threatens the social fabric. Thus, Berger writes,[19] "Every socially constructed nomos must face the constant possibility of its collapse into anomy." Social order, of whatever specific sort in whichever society, is an arena of meaning, patterns of expectations, organization, and basic values—i.e. a *cosmos.* For Berger and the received view, this cosmos is carved out of "a vast mass of meaninglessness"—i.e. *chaos*—"a small clearing of lucidity in a formless, dark, always ominous jungle."

I do not wish here to raise any objections to the received view. I want only to voice a puzzler, something the standard view of play seems unable to accommodate.

Douglas Spaulding, the twelve-year-old boy in Ray Bradbury's enchanting novel *Dandelion Wine*,[20] seems to encounter just what Berger has described when, falling behind his running friends at play, he pauses at the edge of the ravine—Bradbury's powerful image for the "formless, dark, always ominous jungle" of chaos and anomy. Douglas is struck in this moment at the edge of civilization, and he muses: "Who could say where town or wilderness began?" The constant struggle between the civilized and the wild, cosmos and chaos, seemed to reveal to him that the "towns never really won," for "they merely existed in calm peril, fully accoutered with lawn mower, bug spray, and hedge shears, swimming steadily as long as civilization said to swim, but each house ready to sink in green tides, buried forever, when the last man ceased and his trowels and mowers shattered to cereal flakes of rust."[21]

He is momentarily stunned into silence by this dread vision at the edge of the ravine. Yet, it is of no small consequence to note something quite odd and suggestive just at this point. What breaks the vision and returns him to himself—during marginal situations, including his own serious illness and being near death—is *play* and *magic*.

The boys play, even at night in one memorable scene, within the very maw of the ravine. There is a fanciful "happiness machine" which never quite works but is only playful despite Mr. Auffman's efforts to make it "work"; there is the melodic talk of old, old Colonel Freeleigh conjuring roguish visions of the "way things used to be." And, finally, there is the junk-man, Mr. Jonas, who gives Doug the enigmatic, playful, yet healing bottles of air when Doug seems suffocatingly near death: "GREEN DUSK FOR DREAMING BRAND PURE NORTHERN AIR," reads the label of one; the other holds wind from the Aran Isles and Dublin Bay "with salt in it and a strip of flannel fog from the coast of Ireland."[22]

Whatever he passed on, it seems to me the same as what David Rabin brought to mind in his response to me. But over against that is the standard view of play and social order. It is surely a powerful view. It unerringly and with elegance expresses what is unmistakably the central view of modern social science: the human career is an earnest path of maturation out of the childish frolics of youth to the resolute seriousness of the adult's social order, whose sheltering quality shields against the terrors of the night: senselessness and lurking disorder. For this view, of course, social life, however stable its nomic form, is always precarious and inwardly threatened by the cunning guises of the formless, the caprice and hazards of bodily life, and the unspeakable madness of the ominous, foreboding clutches of the meaningless. In *Dandelion Wine*, it is The Lonely One, who speaks out of the ravine at night (always at night) to ambush the unwary, to catch us all in our ultimate vulnerability and defenselessness, and who shoves us rudely into the dark ravine of dread, madness, and death. Social life, as sheltering nomos, gives us grounds on which to stand and take our bearings; The Lonely One strips us of these, opens up the abyss with no ground, no holds, no footing with which to take our bearings.

All this seems clearly the texturing quality of the

accident of illness or injury, of the capricious, unfair, unaccountable way we are struck down by disease or wounds. The received view of social life and play gives the basic meaning to the painful, besetting question "Why me?" even while there simply is no way in which that view can answer that searing question.

And yet, David Rabin asks: "Why *not* me?" In our daily lives, as in *Dandelion Wine*, but by no means in the standard social scientific view, we...play, at times sportively, at times defiantly. At the very brink, at the edge of the ravine, we game it up, we frolic and defy the ravine; we cavort, run and sing, muscle one another and cut a jig at death. We enchant and amuse each other with jokes, sometimes cutting jibes, at our afflictions and handicaps ("That's pretty good for a cripple," the character Harrison is told by an attendant). Baffled and staggered though we may be at times, we conjure meaning from magical bottles and monkeyshine, we romp and tickle, disport ourselves with games and wit. With reels and rigadoons, escapades and antics, we flaunt and chortle to the very end.

Against this, even the Lonely One turns out to be witless and impotent. "Why *not* me?" Who can gainsay that ironic twist? How can we reckon with this mummery in the face of the tight-fitting nomos of social life and gaping jaws of chaos, as seen in the dominant view of play and culture? What can we make of that oddly soaring quality of play, and how terribly right it somehow seems, even when it also seems so inappropriate? Pascal, for all his incredible insights, still lamented how we inadvertently "play the lute and dance" instead of grappling with our condition with the earnestness it demands. Kierkegaard, too, was stunned by the oddity of the way people treat the finite with infinite care yet give the infinite only finite, passing glances.

Viewed from the received perspective, such playfulness must seem wholly out of place, mere useless and immature (if not pathological) playing around. David Rabin *must* be at least a bit unbalanced, even clinically depressed, if only momentarily; for one with his remarkable alertness and intelligence could not possibly say to his own dreadful disease, "Why *not* me?" Despair and lamentation seem most in order when the social order is breeched by suffering, illness, or loss—certainly not merriment and play.

The philosopher Susanne Langer[23] once acidly remarked, commenting on the view that the human mind is really nothing but the brain and learns to function simply in the interests of the biological needs which current genetic psychology and biomedicine postulate and recognize: "It seems poor economy of nature that men will suffer and starve for the sake of play, when play is supposed to be the abundance of their strength after their needs are satisfied." The received view makes it hard if not impossible to reckon with the insistent presence of playfulness, for rather than either disappearing or being transformed, it clearly continues throughout life in spite of the growth of rules and codes. It often stupefies our comprehension by cropping up in the supposedly most dreadful of circumstances. There is still that soaring, cleansing, releasing element even in the most organized forums of social life.

With his characteristic genius for fastening onto the essential, but at times with maddening brevity, the Spanish philosopher, Jose Ortega y Gasset, picks up on just this oddly soaring element manifested by play. He notes how the evolution of living creatures is in fact marked by sheer abundance and exuberance, even caprice. "Each species builds up its stock of useful habits by selecting among, and taking advantage of, the innumerable useless actions which a living being performs out of sheer exuberance."[24] The physician Bernard Towers has also observed that "we should look on nature as constantly in motion, trying everything possible, and for the most part at random: 'groping,' as the process was described by Teilhard de Chardin, or 'tinkering,' as Francois Jacob recently put it. Natural selection does not work as an engineer works. It works like a tinkerer—a tinkerer who does not know exactly what he is going to produce but uses whatever he finds around him...living organisms are historical structures; literally creations of history. They represent not a perfect product of engineering, but a patchwork of odd sets pieced together when and where opportunities arose."[25]

As Ortega views organic phenomena, they fall into one of two large classes of activity or effort: "one original, creative, vital par excellence...; the other of utilitarian character, in which the first is put to use and mechanized."[26] The latter puts to use and routinizes what the first spontaneously invents without an eye on utility. The vital force he identifies as *play*, "sportive activity, the foremost and creative, the most exalted, serious, and important part of life." The other, expressed best by labor and work, "is derivative and precipitate. Nay more, life, properly speaking, resides in the first alone; the rest is relatively mechanic (i.e. routine) and a mere functioning." The second, of course, whether in the form of work, social roles, or institutional rules, in its turn may provide the occasion for further playful inventiveness and ingenuity: so-called "bending the rules," or finding new ways for fulfilling typified routines "to make things more interesting," for instance. Life, Ortega urges, "is an affair of flutes. It is overflow that it needs most.... Life has triumphed on this planet because it has, instead of clinging to necessities, deluged it with overwhelming possibilities, so that the failure of one may serve as a bridge for the victory of another."

Here, as with Berger, Ortega clearly endorses the idea that culture, human life, takes shape within the context of biological givens. But how different is the understanding of biology and biological evolution! For what Berger takes to be biological *necessities*, Ortega (along with Towers and evolutionists like Jacob) argues with considerable evidence and insight are *possibilities*. What for the standard view are stable, relatively rigid givens, for Ortega are sportive, playful, and always creative "tinkerings" and exuberant inventions.

The same critical difference emerges regarding human society. Where the received view, essentially a cautious conservatism, posits the social order of rules, roles, codes, and laws as "a sheltering shield" against the terror of anomy, Ortega to the contrary emphasizes that more basic than that merely derivative form of activity is the creative, spontaneous, energetic, and restless striving and play of life in its most exalted form. The standard view's stress is on mere routine, the functionally utilitarian; Ortega's is on the ingenuity and sportiveness which produces in the first place what then may become routinized.

And, regarding the individual within any culture, there is the same crucial difference. The received view sees the individual basically as the creature of culture and society, as nurtured and sheltered against risk and danger which threatens the social order and therefore the individual. The individual who breaks or is broken from the social nomos stands naked in the abyss: without grounds, bearings, meaning, or values. The individual's proper career and destiny is work, adherence to the norms of culture, working within the rules and routines of society. Precisely in this respect, that view commits the fundamental error, for it mistakes the vital impulse of exuberant life for mere childish playing-around; it mistakes the creative play of overflowing, spontaneous life for the merely derivative, merely functional forms of human life. In a word, it mistakes possibility for necessity, and thus cannot comprehend the very nature of play, therefore of human culture and biological evolution more generally. With Doug in *Dandelion Wine* and Ben Harrison in *Whose Life Is It Anyway?*, the basic impulse of human life is to cut a jig and crack a joke in the face of the risks and hazards being human entails, and thereby alone to preserve the full reality of human dignity.

With wonderful directness, Ortega hits upon the crucial clue of that elusive phenomenon nestled in David Rabin's otherwise only curious, and possibly crazy, response "Why *not* me?" It is here, I think, that we find not only the pulse of life's magic, humor, and central beat, but something about life that is wholly absorbing: that it is self-endorsing and inherently valuable. Here, as in no other phenomenon, is what it means to be a *moral* being. Gabriel Marcel,[27] seeking to grasp the oddly fragile yet vigorous sinew of human life, calls it "the exclamatory consciousness of existing"—the emphatic declaration "I am!" It is that ebullient yet enigmatic sense of being alive that Doug[28] comes upon while wrestling with his younger brother: "I'm alive, I'm *really* alive!" he thought. "I never knew it before, or if I did I don't remember!"

That aliveness, whose fullest metaphor is that exclamation point of self-discovery, is a fabric with an unmistakable sense of "worth." Its native air is the rich field of play among the possibles inherent to life. Most fundamentally, I believe, it is the moral order in its clearest form. This vital impulse of play, surely, may well become ensnared in the niggling webs of worry about the necessary and the useful; a person may, suddenly or slowly exposed to the debilitating realities of illness or injury, find himself confronted with the abyss, outside the routines and rules of the accepted social order. He or she may then be in dread. "Why me?"

It is this aliveness, too, which is often diminished, flagged, and afflicted in serious illness—weakened and waning as alertness also fades. But this sense of aliveness may also crop out, always unexpectedly it seems, in new exuberance and invention, sometimes in anger and at times in unaccountable joy. It may flower and dance in the career of a people or in that of a person. It is just this sense of aliveness which, despite the dozy camouflage of the social nomos, despite the utilitarian fixation on rules and norms, shines out unerringly in the play of children, the games of youth, and the sports of adults. It shines out, too, in the words of David Rabin.

What is so striking about this vital pulse of play is how pervasive it is, how quickly recognized and valued—quite in spite of the received view's muting of it. However difficult it assuredly is to talk about it, much less to define it with precision, each of us experiences it all the time: in playing a piece of music with "just the right touch" (or, for that matter, when we listen to it done that way); when we pull off a perfect finesse (or witness one); when a speech "comes off" and the audience is "with it"; when we make something ourselves with care and craft (or see one made that way); when something is done "with style" or "flair." Each of us knows full well that soaring feeling, and knows it to be intrinsically worthwhile and significant, something which often makes otherwise dull routine interesting. Despite the eloquence of a Berger, a Piaget, or a Mead, something is deeply askew therein: the view distorts, and even obfuscates, what is so essential and worthwhile about human life.

But the standard view is both dominant and powerful. Indeed, far beyond its place at the forefront of social science, L.D. Kliever suggests,[29] it is the dominant view of our culture as a whole. It provides the major ways in which science, medicine, law, religion, and other major cultural formations are to be understood and sustained. The "tragic irony of modern religious consciousness," he in effect contends, is that while the heart of all religion is the drama of the meeting of God and man—called by van der Leeuw "holy play"—precisely this vital, creative impulse has been either denigrated to a form of mere immaturity, or commercialized into the irrelevance of a leisure pastime. It is thus no accident that we fear death and illness, loss and suffering—and go to the extremes of concealment and denial which David Rabin found all around him so acutely. In Kliever's uncommonly insightful terms: "Faced with the finality of death, we may respond in two ways. We may 'rage, rage, against the dying of the light' or we may 'play, play, against the coming of the night.' The first is the mandate for all science. The search for knowledge is the heroic quest for the extension of life—it is rage against the dying of the light. The second response is the heart of all religion. The venture of faith is the heroic quest of the enhancement of life—it is play against the coming of the night."

I would add to this but one observation. The "rage" which is the mandate for all science seems especially prominent in biomedical science and medicine. As the social order is, for the standard view, a "shield against terror," modern medicine is the crucial ally for that view with its centering focus on curing disease and injury, and thus restoring afflicted persons to normal membership in the social order. Those who, like David Rabin, cannot be "cured" thus not only stand outside medicine as beyond its apparent powers, but also are living affronts to it. Being "incurable" is being "beyond help," and this all too easily becomes the motive for being *abandoned*. The incurable stands outside not only medicine, but often outside the concerns of the social world and its presumed "shelter," and thus confronts the rest of us with the stark terror of meaninglessness.

For the received view, the question asked by many patients—"Why me?"—presents a crucial catch-22: while it seems the only understandable, if not reasonable, question when disaster strikes, it is yet utterly unanswerable. "Why me?" is the same as asking, "Why has the social shelter failed to shield me against this terror?"

But the response of David Rabin—"Why *not* me?"— is far, far different, for it is a rejection of the very framework of the received view of things. It says, I have suggested, with Ortega, that life has not ceased, that vitality and exuberance are not only still with him, but are the genuine reality; it says that "play" is the most exalted and serious aspect of life. David Rabin's response, that elusively playful "Why not?" is a critical reaffirmation that the only finally significant form of "cure" is "care," and that the finest medicine for an afflicted human being must always include that endorsement of human life by play and its inherently caring presence. To forget this is to forget ultimately what we are.

In response to a conversation about this essay with David and Pauline, I've been reading it again and trying to sharpen the central motif: "Why not me?" as luck would have it—another of the delightful chance occurrences—I received a remarkable letter from a woman, Ms. Kay Toombs, to whom I had sent an earlier version of this essay.[30] Afflicted with multiple sclerosis, she just discovered that she has now developed a constriction of her carotid artery. Her response to the essay is both more eloquent and clearer than I could hope to achieve. Writing of serious illness as a kind of "sentence" and an example of the "extreme capriciousness of fate," she poignantly suggests how the received view of the social order not only forces the "Why me?" experience, but thereby greatly adds to the burden of illness. "The 'Why me?' focuses only on the arbitrariness and unfairness of the personal situation. It imprisons one within the chaos. It destroys the ability to retain a meaningful existence.... It implies that... the individual is not only not whole in body, but also somehow fragmented in spirit."

Yet, she writes, "Strangely enough, like David Rabin, I found myself asking the different question, 'Why *not* me?'—and I found this to be a strangely liberating question. In a sense, it removed the overwhelming feeling of victimization, of being singled out. I further found myself asking, 'And if *not* me, why someone else?' " As she writes, this question "puts things back into a certain perspective. It reminds one of the radical contingency of existence in all its aspects. In a real way it frees one from the eternal torment of the 'Why me?'...Why *not* me? *No* reason. And, since there is no reason, I am free to put the question aside—and to go from there. This is, for sure, a liberation."

Only play, she insists, enables us to deal with the capriciousness of fate and what it doles out willy-nilly. "It is the means to preserve the integrity of the spirit within. It is our way of declaring that we are still the same person—even if our physical body has changed.... To accept that playfulness as not only appropriate but as something to be nurtured and cultivated seems to me to be extremely important—rather than something to be decried or written off as slightly pathological. It is, indeed, the very essence of caring, and, in a sense, of 'curing.' One can 'survive' anything, if one can retain a sense of humor. Without it, one is trapped."

As I said, I don't know any way to improve on these reflections. This woman, from within her own grievously afflicted condition, not only shares the same insight as David Rabin but points unerringly to the very core of what makes us moral beings: "And if *not* me, why somebody else?" What she reports as so powerfully liberating is not only being released from the sense of victimization, but thereby being enabled to relate to other persons and their plights. For the received view, to the contrary, morality and ethics can only be an affair of rules whose character is ultimately denial: part of the nomic cast of rules designed merely to shelter, protect, against the dying of the light. It is in this both basically pointless and blind to the very rudiments of our human condition, our mortality and vulnerability. As a denial and refusal to face our common condition, ethics so understood is in effect a way, however subtle, of constricting each of us and limiting our vision to ourselves. It is a way of refusing to recognize other persons, and thus of persuading us that we are abandoned and alone.

On the other hand, her words insistently remind us that when we focus on the soaring and playful elements in human life, moral life and ethics are transformed into a positive embracing of our common humanity and the thrust of life seeking to nurture it in all ways, to cultivate the fields of the possible and enable them to become actual. Play is an exercise in the *imaginational*, as is morality. Thus, play and creativity must be recognized as the center of all education, moral education especially: the tending to and enabling, hence freeing, of the vital drama of human life—even, or especially when facing loss, suffering, illness, and death. It may be that only play, in all its rich variety, can cure; certainly, it alone can care.

Thank you, David, for upsetting me, thus caring.

References

1. Zaner, R.M. Chance and morality: the dialysis phenomenon. In: *The Humanity of the Ill: Phenomenological Perspectives*, Kestenbaum V. (ed.). Knoxville, Tenn.: University of Tennessee Press, 1982, pp. 39-68.

2. Spiegelberg, H. Accident of birth: a non-utilitarian motif in Mill's philosophy. *J. Hist. Ideas* 22:475-492, 1961.

3. Foster, L. Man and machine: life without kidneys. *Hastings Cancer Rep.* 6:6-8, 1976.

4. Spiegelberg, H., op. cit.

5. Spiegelberg, H. A defense of human equality. *Philos. Rev.* 53:101-24, 1944.

6. Spiegelberg, H. Good fortune obligates: Albert Schweitzer's second ethical principal. *Ethics* 85:227-34, 1975.

7. Spiegelberg, H. Ethics for fellows in the fate of existence. In: *Mid-Twentieth Century American Philosophy*, Bertocci, P.A. (ed.). New York: Humanities Press, 1974, pp. 193-210.

8. Spiegelberg, H. Human dignity: a challenge to contemporary philosophy. *Philos. Forum* 9:39-64, 1971.

9. Spiegelberg, H. A defense of human equality. Op. cit.

10. Spiegelberg, H. Good fortune obligates. Op. cit.

11. Ibid.

12. Beaumont, C. Hair of the dog. In: *Yonder*, Beaumont, C. (ed.). New York: Bantam Books, Inc., 1958, pp. 121-133.

13. Piaget, J. *The Origins of Intelligence in Children*, Cook, M. (tr.). New York: International Universities Press, 1952.

14. Mead, G.H. *Mind, Self and Society*. Chicago: The University of Chicago Press, 1934.

15. Piaget, J. *Play, Dreams and Imitation in Childhood*, Hodgson, F.M. (tr.). New York: W.W. Norton Company, 1962.

16. Mead, G.H., op. cit.

17. Berger, P. *The Sacred Canopy: Elements of a Sociological Theory of Religion*. Garden City, N.Y.: Doubleday, Anchor Books, 1969.

18. Jaspers, K. *General Psychopathology*. Chicago: University of Chicago Press, 1963.

19. Berger, P., Op. cit.

20. Bradbury, R. *Dandelion Wine*. New York: Bantam Books, 1956.

21. Ibid.

22. Ibid.

23. Langer, Susanne. *Philosophy in a New Key*. New York: New American Library, 1942.

24. Ortega y Gasset, J. *History as a System, and Other Essays Toward a Philosophy of History*. New York: W.W. Norton Company, 1961, pp. 16-21.

25. Towers, B. The origin and development of living forms. *J. Med. Philos*. 1:88-106, 1978.

26. Ortega y Gasset, J., op. cit.

27. Marcel, G. *De Mystere de l'etre*, t. I: *Reflexion et mystere*. Paris: Aubier, Editions Montaigne, 1951.

28. Bradbury, R., op. cit.

29. Kliever, L.D. Polysymbolism and modern religiosity. *J. Religion* 59:169-194, 1979.

30. Passages from Ms. Kay Toombs letter (of August 16, 1983) are used with her kind permission (letter of August 28, 1983).

Index

A

Abnormal development, no cause for alarm, 144
Addicted patient, drug abuse in, 112
A.L.S., 29, 31, 38, 39, 43, 48, 49, 51, 226
Alzheimer's disease, 49, 136
Ambiguity, dealing with, 199
Amniocentesis, 162
Analgesic adjuncts, 114
Analgesics, administration of, 113
  narcotic, 112
Anger, 43, 58, 59, 63, 65, 66, 70, 75, 76, 77, 78, 158
  healthy, expressions of, 77, 78
  nothing to do with people who are target, 173
Anxiety, 6, 10, 19, 23, 45, 66, 82, 87, 100, 103, 111, 122, 129, 150, 181
  physicians', 128
Assessment of function, opportunities for intervention, 138

B

Behavioral treatment techniques, 139
Bereavement, 105
Biopsychosocial model, 119
Body image, loss of, 83
Busy physician, time to sit down by patient's bed, 197

C

Cancer, 65, 70, 71, 73, 74, 76, 82, 84
  battle lost to, 69

center, 66
diagnosis of, 82
fear of intractable pain, 109
I hate having, 77
likelihood of pain, 110
live with, 89
living alongside of, 91
patient dying of, 82
patients, 66, 68, 69, 75, 82
  human rights of, 77
  image of, 76
victims, 69, 76
Cancer patient,
  families of, 85
  management of, 88
  physician's reactions to, 86
  physician's role for, 90
Care,
  of the demented, changes, 134
  patient-family, 101
  quality of, 81
Career in medicine, self-evaluation, 215
Caring physician,
  education of, 202
  nurturing sides of, 134
Chaos and anomy, 231
Chemotherapy, 42, 54, 55-58, 61, 62, 64
  lessons of, 63
Choices, 74
Clinical picture, xviii, 5, 24
Coming to terms, 71
Commitment to science and humanism, 214
Communication, failure of, 60

Communications, discouraged, 129
Compassion, xvii
  acquisition of, 214
  and humanism to students, importance of role modeling, 214
  reach out to the poor, 215
Computerized information, 24
Concern, 68
  lack of, 67
  sustained, 35
Control, 87, 93
  loss of, 83
Coping mechanisms, 61, 64
Crises, 62
Curing and caring, 80, 178
Curiosity, morbid, 56

D

Death,
  accepted without fear, 168
  as a forbidden subject, 169
  attitudes toward, 167
    shameful and forbidden, 168
  children not exposed to, 169
  classifications of, 81
  difficulty coping with, 169
  interdict of, 45
  medical-biologic model, 94
  news imparted by physician involved in care, 188
  news presented in clear manner, 188
  state of, 81
  the acceptance process, 170

understanding of, 81
Western attitudes toward, 168
Death sentence, 66
Decisions, made with patient's interests in mind, 218
Definitive therapy, 30
Demented patient(s),
 care of, 133
 cognitive function as objective, 137
 dismissed by physicians, 136
 function-oriented approach, 138
 human needs, 136
 physician's sense of mission, 137
 physician's role,
  to fight the disease of, 136
  who would care for, 136
 readjustment in attitudes toward, 137
 shunned by physicians, 134
Dementia, 134
 diagnosis of depression, 139
 reversible disorders, 135
 modified by treatment, 135
Denial, 82, 84
 by medical caretaker, 144
 dealing with, 90
 duty to help patient face reality, 172
 is hope, 91
Dependency, 83
 increasing, 89
Depersonalizing effect, 66

Depression, 68, 75, 100, 103, 111, 181
 anticipation of what is to come, 175
 a second illness, 128
 reaction to illness, 175
 treatment of, 89
Diagnosis, reactions to, 85
Discrimination, 75
Disease,
 chronic, 46
  devotion of physician to, 200
 combatant against, 133
 hateful, free of, 70
 intellectualizing about, 84
Disease process, xviii
Doctor, avoidance or denial reactions, 199
Doctor-patient relationship, complaints about, 201
Dying, 81
 acceptance, 176
 anger, 172
 a public event, 168
 bargaining, 173
 denial, 171
 depressive, 174
 determining right time to prolong life, 178
 exposure to, 45
 family needs more help than patient, 177
 five stages, 171
 patient allowed to express sorrow, 175
 preparation for death, 179
 process of, 94

treatment of depressions, 175
why me, 172
Dying patient(s), xviii, 25, 81
be there for, 183
dyspnea, 180
difficulties in dealing with, 86
mental anguish, 181
social pain, 181

E

Education, effect on attitude, 121
Educational goals, 129
Emotion(s)
and cancer patients, 64, 76
influence on disease of, 18
in physicians, attitude toward mental illness, 128
paralysis of, 82
psychoneurotic reactions and, 9, 10
states of, 6, 25
stimuli to, 12
stress caused by, 100
survival of, 61
Empathy, 130
Encouragement, important therapy for A.L.S., 52
Endorphins, 113
Exercise, 62
Existentialism, 73
Explanations, inadequate, 55

F

Faculty, development of human qualities in students, 219
Failure, feelings of, 59
Family support, 37
Family support system, 139
Fasiculation, 31
Fears, 65, 66, 77, 82, 181
illogical, 70
of the unknown, 82
Frustrations, 60, 64, 65, 68, 122
Functional disorders, 14, 18
Functional disturbances, 12, 13, 19, 20
Functional approach, opposition to, 140

G

Genetic counseling,
child affected by chronic disease, 155
communicating diagnosis to new parents, 157
disease in other children, 155
information to other family members, 152
needs of parents, 157
patients, low self-esteem, 150
prenatal diagnosis, 155
question of reproduction, 155

risk factors, 151
the affected child, 155
the affected fetus, 161
the affected newborn, 157
understanding emotional
  needs, 150
Genetic disease,
  the affected adult, 153
  concerns about, 150
  preclinical detection, 154
  prevention of occurrence,
  160
Genetic diagnosis, self-image,
154
Genetic disorders, immediate
  care of child, 158
Grief, 33, 85, 86, 158, 165
  acute, 186
  administrative concerns,
  189
  alarm, 186
  ambiance of emergency
  room, 189
  anger, 187
  anxiety, 187
  chief mourner, 189
  crisis intervention, 191
  fight or flight response, 186
  immediate phase,
    management of, 188
    reactions, 186
    three clinical patterns,
    186
  management of,
    general principles, 188
    special considerations,
    189

medication, 190
  staff reaction, 191
Grief reaction, 185
  three phases, 186
Guilt, 72, 75, 82, 83, 85, 90,
101, 122, 150
  feelings of, 158
  mode of transmission, 150,
  151
  replacement by scorn, 122

H

Healing process, 68
Handicapped children, information to help patient and
  family, 145
Health-care workers, reactions to their own mortality, 55
Helpless, 61-64
Helpless feeling, 60
Helplessness, difficulty in
  dealing with, 57
Heroic therapy, 159
Hope, 84
Hospice, 97
  ability to pay, 106
  care,
    Medicare payment plan,
    106
    role of nursing, 104
  goals, reasonable quality
  of life for patient, 102
  interdisciplinary care, 101
  movement, 47

needs of family members,
101
patient and family, 100
peaceful and secure envi-
ronment, 104
primary unit-of-care, 100
program, characteristics, 98
staff support and com-
munication, 105
symptom control, 102
understanding of situation,
101
volunteers, 106
Hospital(s), 66
depersonalize doctor-pa-
tient relationship, 198
for profit, 27
inhospitality of, 68
medical care in, rising
charges, 196
practice, 3
system, 68, 69
teaching, 66
How to tell, 92
Humane physician, qualities,
214
Humanism, 22, 133
in medicine, 170
day of high technology,
210
major concerns, 213
Humanistic medicine, interfere with, 89
Humanity, xvii
Human life, chance in, 223
Human responses, that interfere with care of patient,
217

I

Identity, loss of, 83
If not me, why somebody
else, 242
Illness,
chronic, 43, 60, 61
coping with, 60
incurable, 31, 40
diagnosis of, 80
physician to advise about
ways of living with, 200
Information release, 119
Insecurity, 66
Institutional care, 46
Intellectual function, preservation of, 49
Intractable pain,
management of, 109
double tragedy, 109
Isolation, xiv, xviii, 20, 33,
34, 41, 43, 45, 49, 181
for the patient, 165

K

Knowledge, serious deficiencies of, 121

L

Language of oncology, frightening, 93
Legacy, courage and concern,
75
Life and death situations, 218
Living and dying, decisions
regarding, 213

Loss, 83
Lost function, family unaware of, 139
Love and concern, expressions of, 66
Lymphoma, 55

M

Macular degeneration, 32
Make today count, 76, 77
Manic behavior, 35
Marfan's syndrome, 42
Mass in mid-neck, 54
Medical care,
   cost efficiency, 197
   cost of, 26
Medical education, xvii
   balance between technical competence, professionalism and humane behavior, 205
   classic works of literature, 203
   emphasis on scientific medicine, 195
   historical orientation, 204
   reflections on, 194
   skills in dealing with chronically ill, 205
   social science, 204
   sustain sensitivity and humaneness, 204
   time with the patient, 206
   well-rounded liberal education, 202
Medical education system, role model, 196

Medical insurance, 44
Medical practice, 2
   in hospital, 198
Medications, causing impairment of function, 139
Medicine,
   art of, 3, 94
      communication, 216
   career in, self-evaluation, 215
   divisions into specialties, 195
   practice of, 1-3, 21
   science of, 3
Mental illness
   and psychiatric referral, 126
   and real medicine, 125
   as an action, 123
   as immoral states, 123
   attitude toward, reactions to suicide, 122
   equated with badness or sinfulness, 125
   equated with weakness, 123
   meaning of, 123
   physician's attitude toward, 115
   physician's preparation to cope with, 121
   willpower to overcome symptoms, 125
Mental retardation
   attitude towards, 144
   behavior techniques, 147
   concern for parents' well-being, 143
   conspiracy of silence, 146
   dearth of knowledge, 145

diagnosis bereft of hope, 145
diagnosis devastating, 144
grief process, 144
lack of compassion of doctor, 145
learn to live with it, 145
living in a caring home, 148
positive qualities, 148
resources of the community, 146
siblings love and concern, 147
support services, 146
Mourning, 186
Mouth, hygiene of, 180
Municipal hospital, 25

N

Narcotics,
tolerance to euphoria, 112
side effect of obstipation, 112
Needs, patient's personal and human, 133
Nervous reactions, 12
Neurologist, interview with, 144
News of death, impact of, 186
Non-medicinal prescription, danger involved, 124
Nursing homes, 27, 44, 47
Nursing techniques, 16

O

Obliteration of self, 66
Obstacles to change, xiv
Omnipotence, 87
Oncologist, service in the ending period, 94

P

Pain, 67, 71, 81
acute, 103
defined beginning and end, 110
acute and chronic, 110
chronic, 103
circular, 110
"cocktails", 114
control,
monograph on, 115
of physical and psychologic, 102
emotional reaction to, 111
expectant management, 110
hospice regimen, 103
management, consumerism-humanism in, 114
management of terminal, 179
medication, method of delivery, 103
nature of, 103
pathophysiology, new developments in, 113
physical, 179

Painful procedures, to stay alive, 84
Paralysis agitans, 50
Pariah, 38, 41
Passport of the healthy, 41
Patient,
  as a person, 120
  care of, 3, 16, 21-23, 25
    holistic approach, 119
    team concept, 211
  concerns,
    isolation, 165
    loss of dignity, 165
    pain, 165
  depersonalize, 23
  emotions experienced by, 165
  life of, optimize quality of, 49
  not actually demented, 135
  personality of, 119
  physician's hostility toward, 87
  positive attitude toward psychiatric referral, 127
  practical concerns, 100
  servant to, 133
  terminally ill, 25
  troubles of, physician's emotional distance from, 199
Patient-doctor relationship, 196
Peptic ulcer bleeding, emotional antecedents of, 120
Personal concerns, doctor, 81
Personal identity, 5
Personal problems, patient

confused, 211
Personal relationship, 4, 8, 19, 20, 23
Personalities, cancer-prone, 72
Pharmacologic program, fears of addiction, 102
Philosopher reflects,
  aliveness, 238
  Beaumont, 225
  Berger, 230
  Bradbury, 231
  human society, 236
  individual as creature of culture, 236
  Jacob, 235
  Kliever, 239
  Langer, 234
  Marcel, 237
  Ortega y Gasset, 234-237
  play and culture, 228
  play and magic, 231
  play and seriousness, 227
  Schweitzer, 224
  social conduct, 228
  vital pulse of play, 238
Physical and mental illness, same or different, 118
Physician(s),
  aims of, care of the patient, 137
  as patient, xiv
  alcoholic, 35
  attitude of, information supplied by psychiatrist, 127
  busy, time to sit down by patient's bed, 197

caring nurturing sides of, 134

dual personality of, 212

family, 81

failings, inability to acknowledge limits of expertise, 216

favorable attitude toward psychiatry, 122

feelings of impotence, 137

function of, actively listening, 93

inability to deal with ambiguity, 201

necessary to be available, 202

need to be loved, 87

obligation of, when patient refuses specific treatment, 93

-oncologist, 80

personality of, 128

prolong act of dying, 178

two major roles, 133

uncomfortable with closeness, 87

what do we expect in, 212

who become patients, problems, 55

Physiologic activity, disturbances of, 10

Place of death, hospital or nursing home, 169

Power, sense of, 74, 87

Pregnancy, risk of birth defect, 161

Premature widow syndrome, 41

Premium on privacy, 44

Process of dying, 94

Professional colleagues, reactions of, 31

Professionals, using research to enhance careers, 147

Pseudodementia, 135

Psychiatry,
    medical student's attitude, 126
    nature of the subject matter, 126
    physician's resistance, 127

Psychological factors, 24

Psychoneuroses, 9

Psychotic thinking, response to medications, 139

Q

Quadraplegia, 48

Quality of care, 81

R

Rage, 79

Regression, 83

Reject help, 84

Relationships,
    effects of my illness on, 31
    shared before, 69

Retarded child, parents need an advocate, 146

Retarded infant, therapy in all instances, 160

Retarded newborn, placement of, 159

Retreat, 75, 76
  need to, 70
Risk, 75
Rules,
  doctor's, 65
  hospital's, 65
  medical team's, 65

S

Safe passage, xviii, 25
Self-esteem, 41, 62
  oncologists', 64
Self-hatred, 75
Self-help groups, 153, 157
Self-pity, 75
Service reductions, the poor
  and unemployed, 197
Sick, segregation of, 44
Sick colleagues, compassion
  toward, 36
Sick people, human needs of,
  220
Sick physicians, 42
  ways colleagues can help,
  34
Sickness and health, alter-
  nating, 64
Side effects, 61-63
  threat of, 57
Skills, in resolving human
  problems, 123
Social contact, 41
Social disease, 38, 62
Social framework, 44
Social life, rupture of, 229
Social nomos, 228
Social order, 228, 230

breech of, 230
Social outcasts, 41
Social roles, 229
Social workers, 26
Sorrow, 158
Spiritual component, 182
Stress, 82, 129
  signs of, 82
Students for medicine, strong
  in science, 212
Suicide, talking with patients
  about, 122
Support, 46, 81
  after end of chemotherapy,
  60
  to patient's family, 165
Support system, 40
Symptoms, 82
  bulbar, 48
  response of "interest", 128
Syndrome, premature widow,
  41

T

Terminal illness (disease),
  problems between patient
  and doctor, 198
  patients feel abandoned by
  physicians, 101
  role of physician, 167
Terminally ill, 69, 80, 81
  demands on family caring
  for, 101
  psychologic and social problems, 100
  use of powerful narcotics,
  102

Therapy, stress of termination of, 58
Tolerance and addiction, problems of, 111
Tolerance, pharmacologic, 112
Traditionalism, xv
Treatment,
    active involvement of patient in, 93
    for the patient, 92
    refusing further, 93

U

Ultrasound techniques, 162

Unfairness, 73
Untouchables, 66
Urbanization, 44

V

Vanderbilt, 30

W

Why me, 70, 71, 74, 225, 227, 233, 240, 241
    four possible answers, 72
Why not me, 74, 226, 227, 233, 237, 240, 241